Speech and Language Assessment for the Bilingual Handicapped

Speech and Language Assessment for the Bilingual Handicapped

Larry J. Mattes, Ph.D.
and
Donald R. Omark, Ph.D.

COLLEGE-HILL PRESS, INC., San Diego, California

College-Hill Press
4284 41st Street
San Diego, California 92105

Library of Congress Cataloging in Publication Data
Mattes, Larry J.
Speech and language assessment for the bilingual handicapped

Bibliography: p.
Includes indexes.
1. Speech disorders in children. 2. Language disorders in children. 3. Bilingualism. 4. Physically handicapped children—Language. I. Omark, Donald R. II. Title.
RJ 496.S7M38 1984 618.92'855 84-9601.
ISBN 0-933014-01-5

Printed in the United States of America

DEDICATION

This book is dedicated to speech–language pathologists and all other professionals who are making an effort to improve current practices in the assessment of children from bilingual, bicultural backgrounds.

CONTENTS

Dedication, v

Contents, vii

Preface and Acknowledgments, ix

Chapter 1 Assessing the Bilingual Child: Differences versus Disorders, 1

Chapter 2 Developing a Bilingual Assessment Team, 17

Chapter 3 Roles for Professionals in Assessment, 31

Chapter 4 Assessing Cultural and Environmental Influences, 41

Chapter 5 Published Tests and Their Limitations, 53

Chapter 6 Alternatives to Standardized Language Tests, 71

Chapter 7 Modifying and Constructing Assessment Instruments, 89

Chapter 8 Educational Program Planning, 105

Appendix A Guidelines for Interviewing Parents About Cultural and Environmental Influences, 111

Appendix B Test Descriptions and Publishers' Addresses, 113

Appendix C Test Evaluation Form, 127

Appendix D Characteristics of Minority Languages Spoken in the United States, 131

Appendix E Exercises, 141

References, 143

Author Index, 155

Subject Index, 159

PREFACE

One of the urgent challenges faced by speech–language pathologists working in school settings is that of developing effective strategies for the assessment and identification of bilingual children with communicative disorders. Traditionally, the responsibility for administering tests* to children with suspected communicative disorders has been that of the speech–language pathologist. However, often the speech–language pathologist does not speak the child's language and/or there are no appropriate test instruments available. The supply of bilingual speech–language pathologists is insufficient to meet the needs of Spanish-speaking children and all of the other language minority groups attending our schools. Moreover, few training programs in the field of speech–language pathology offer coursework designed to train students to work with bilingual student populations. Thus, many practicing speech–language pathologists are inadequately prepared for roles in the assessment of bilingual children.

Because of the shortage of bilingual speech–language pathologists and test instruments in languages other than English, children from bilingual, bicultural backgrounds are often not assessed when a disorder is suspected. Many teachers are hesitant to refer bilingual children for speech–language assessments because of the shortage of appropriately qualified assessment personnel. Some speech–language pathologists see little point in trying to identify communicatively handicapped bilingual children because the local school district has made no effort to provide remedial services in any language other than English.

Action must be taken to meet the needs of communicatively handicapped bilingual children even if the services of a bilingual speech–language pathologist cannot be obtained. The consequence of doing nothing is a loss of services to children who need special attention. Failure to provide communicatively handicapped children with remedial services reduces the likelihood that these children will experience success within the educational curriculum.

If bilingual children with communicative disorders are to be appropriately identified, a team approach is needed. Thus, speech–language pathologists need to work closely with professionals from other disciplines and with bilingual members of the community in all aspects of the assessment process. Moreover, they have to participate in the development of programs designed to train bilingual personnel for roles in assessment.

Speech and Language Assessment for the Bilingual Handicapped is intended to meet the needs of school personnel concerned about improving current practices in the speech and language assessment of children from bilingual,

*The term *test,* as used in this book, refers to any procedure, standardized or nonstandardized, that is used in assessment to examine specific aspects of the child's behavior.

bicultural backgrounds. In addition to presenting a review of issues in the identification of communicatively handicapped bilingual children, this book details specific guidelines for developing an appropriate assessment battery for local use, implementing a team approach to assessment, training assessment personnel, and conducting the testing in a nondiscriminatory manner. The importance of assessing communication within a pragmatic framework is emphasized throughout the text.

In writing this book, an attempt has been made to avoid the excessive use of complex linguistic terminology so that the content can be understood by members of the assessment team who do not have extensive training in the field of speech–language pathology. Thus, the information presented in this book should be useful to monolingual and bilingual speech–language pathologists, school psychologists, bilingual education teachers, and others who may be asked to participate in various aspects of the assessment process. If the content of this book proves to be of practical value in the speech and language assessment of bilingual children, then our purpose will have been accomplished.

Larry J. Mattes
Academic Communication Associates
P.O. Box 6044
Oceanside, CA 92056

Donald R. Omark
Los Amigos Research Associates
7035 Galewood
San Diego, CA 92120

ACKNOWLEDGMENTS

We express our gratitude to those who assisted in the review of the manuscript and offered suggestions that were helpful in the writing of this book. Barbara Hodson, Rhonda Johnson, Gene Ramos, George Santiago, Kathlyn Thompson, and Daniel Watson each provided valuable assistance. We also thank College-Hill Press for publishing a book in which assessment procedures are described that are somewhat nontraditional and outside the mainstream of current assessment practices.

Chapter 1

Assessing the Bilingual Child: Differences Versus Disorders

The use of tests in the identification of handicapped children from bilingual, bicultural backgrounds is one of the most politically sensitive issues in the field of special education today. In the past, children whose primary language was not English often were misidentified as handicapped and placed in special education programs based on the results of tests administered in English and biased in favor of the Anglo middle class population (Mercer, 1980, 1983). Court cases in which the use of these tests was challenged have had a major impact on policies relating to the assessment of minority group children (Oakland & Laosa, 1977).

The development of nonbiased procedures for the assessment of bilingual, bicultural children has become a major concern among special educators since passage of the Education for All Handicapped Children Act (Public Law 94-142) in 1975. This law contains provisions requiring that testing be conducted in a nondiscriminatory manner, using assessment procedures that are culturally and linguistically appropriate. Placement in special education programs is appropriate only for children with specific handicaps that require a *remedial* program. Second language learners who perform poorly in the school setting because of limited familiarity with English and/or cultural differences need to be distinguished from children who demonstrate communicative disorders and/or other abnormalities that require special education intervention.

A comprehensive speech–language assessment is essential when testing is conducted to determine the educational needs of bilingual, bicultural individuals with suspected handicaps. Educational psychologists, specialists in learning disabilities, and others involved in the assessment of academic and intellectual functioning need to know what language problems, if any, may be contributing to the child's poor school performance. The speech–language pathologist is likely to be called upon to provide this information.

The identification of communicatively disordered bilingual children is difficult, especially when the speech–language pathologist speaks only English.

BILINGUALISM AND COMMUNICATIVE DISORDERS

The term *bilingual*, as used in this book, refers to individuals who have been exposed to two languages in natural speaking contexts and who come from homes where they have made functional use of a language other than that of the dominant culture during interactions with one or more family members. We view bilingualism as existing on a continuum, with monolingualism at one end and nativelike fluency in two languages at the other (Kachru, 1965; see McCollum, 1981).

In the speech and language assessment of bilingual, bicultural children, *communicative differences* that are typical of individuals learning a second language must be distinguished from *communicative disorders*. A disorder is present when speaking behavior is defective to such an extent that it interferes with one's ability to convey messages clearly and effectively during interactions with community members who speak the same language and dialect. A limited English proficient child should not be considered to have a speech or language disorder if the "problems" observed reflect the child's limited experiences in using the English language.

When children who speak English as a second language are referred for speech–language evaluations, procedures are needed to ensure that testing is conducted in the native language. Assessment personnel must become sensitive to the complex factors involved in the identification of bilingual children with disorders of *voice, fluency, articulation,* and *language*.

VOICE DISORDERS

Voice disorders include abnormalities in vocal quality (e.g., hoarseness, breathiness, hypernasality), pitch, and/or intensity. Abnormalities in voice production should be judged from a criterion of vocal hygiene and also in terms of acoustical and cultural standards (Perkins, 1971). Cultural groups can be expected to differ in the esthetic standards used to judge the adequacy of voice production. Speech that is judged to be extremely nasal by one culture may be considered normal by another culture (Linares, 1983).

Assessment personnel must recognize that the manner in which vocal quality, pitch, and intensity are used varies from culture to culture. A second language learner should not be considered to have a voice disorder if voice "problems" are observed in English that reflect the influence of *normal* habits of voice production from the first language. A voice disorder is present only if the quality, pitch, and/or intensity of the voice results in a reduction in speech intelligibility or is esthetically unpleasant to members of the child's culture. The most serious consideration, however, is vocal hygiene. Children who demonstrate voice disorders resulting from abuse to the laryngeal mechanism must receive immediate attention.

Moncur and Brackett (1974) recommend that evaluations of vocal functioning include measurements of (1) adequacy of breath for speech, (2) laryngeal valving, (3) behavior of the vibrator, (4) use of the resonators, and (5) prosody characteristics. Specific procedures are suggested by Moncur and Brackett for assessing each of these five aspects of voice production. These procedures can be used with speakers of any language if care is taken to develop stimulus materials (e.g., word lists) that are culturally and linguistically appropriate.

Although voice disorders typically manifest themselves in both languages, it is recommended that limited English proficient children be assessed in their first language. If assessment is conducted only in the second language, vocal behaviors that reflect the influence of normal habits of voice production from the first language may be difficult to distinguish from voice characteristics resulting from a disorder. Therefore, data obtained when limited English proficient children are assessed in their first language are more likely to provide a valid measure of their vocal behavior.

Severe voice disorders such as extreme hoarseness can generally be detected quite easily in either of the child's languages. Children who are found to demonstrate voice disorders should be referred to a physician for evaluation of the laryngeal mechanism. Boone (1971) emphasized that "no patient should receive voice therapy from the speech pathologist unless the voice problem has been diagnosed by a physician competent in the field of laryngology" (p. 72).

FLUENCY DISORDERS

Fluency disorders are characterized by an abnormal rate and/or rhythm of speech. Stuttering, the most common fluency disorder, affects the flow of speech and is characterized by "repetitions or prolongations of a sound, or syllable, or articulatory posture, or by avoidance and struggle reactions" (Van Riper, 1972, p. 249).

Stuttering disorders are often difficult to distinguish from problems reflecting limited proficiency in the language. The following utterances were obtained from the language sample of a 7-year-old Hispanic male who was learning English as a second language:

> Yesterday I go to the store and buy uh uh buy the thing, you know, for the finger. I buy buy the uh buy the ring. My friend come and we play the uh, we play uh, we play the park. And we go to my house.

This child's speech in English was characterized by frequent hesitations and word repetitions, but these problems were not observed in Spanish. The hesitations and word repetitions tended to occur when the child was experiencing an inability to think of the appropriate English word to use to express his thoughts. Thus, the observed behaviors resulted from the individual's limited proficiency in English rather than from a stuttering disorder.

Children learning a first language are often observed to go through a period in which their speech is characterized by frequent dysfluencies (Van Riper, 1972). Second language learners also demonstrate these behaviors as a result of their limited ability to communicate in English. Fluency disorders which are abnormalities in the *rhythm* of speech must not be confused with problems resulting from lack of vocabulary (Linares, 1983).

Bilingual children with suspected stuttering disorders should be assessed in both languages. If dysfluent speech is observed only in English, then it is likely that the problems observed reflect the child's limited proficiency in English. Cases of stuttering disorders in one language and not in the other have been reported (Dale, 1977). Therefore, the careful analysis of the child's communicative behavior in a variety of speaking contexts is essential.

Cultural differences in attitudes toward stuttering are an important factor to consider in determining whether the child has a disorder. In our society, stuttering is viewed as an abnormality and those who stutter are likely to experience frequent social rejection (Van Riper, 1972). In contrast, Lemert (1962) found that Manganians viewed stuttering as an inborn characteristic and did not socially reject those who stuttered. In a study of the problem of stuttering in North American Indian Societies, Stewart (1960) found that the Cowichans often viewed the cause of stuttering as supernatural. Thus, cultural groups differ in the extent to which children are held responsible for their speech fluency. Moreover, cultural groups differ in the extent to which stuttering is viewed as a disability that can be remediated.

ARTICULATION DISORDERS

An articulation disorder is present when the child demonstrates deficits in the production of the speech sounds of the language. Traditionally, speech–language pathologists assessed production of individual phonemes without considering the systematic nature of the observed phonemic inadequacies. The phonological approach to assessment has become popular in recent years. This approach focuses on the examination of the phonological processes used by the child rather than focusing solely on the individual phoneme errors produced. Incorrect production of a particular phoneme may be the result of different phonological processes in different situations. Thus, the specific patterns of error need to be examined (Hodson & Paden, 1983). As a result of recent research findings on phonological processes, investigators have suggested that children diagnosed as having *functional articulation disorders* are better described as having *phonological disorders* (see McReynolds & Elbert, 1981).

Children learning English as a second language often are observed to pronounce English words differently from monolingual English speakers.

Second language learners are faced with the complex task of learning a phonological system that may differ, in many respects, from the phonological system of their native language. Phonological differences that reflect the individual's limited proficiency in English should not be viewed as disorders.

Spanish-speaking children learning English, for example, may be observed to omit particular sounds and to produce substitutions such as *sh* for *ch*, *t* for voiceless *th*, and *d* for voiced *th* (Cairns, Cairns, & Williams, 1974; Cornejo, 1973). There are important differences between the sound systems of English and Spanish that appear to contribute to the problems experienced by Spanish speakers in pronouncing English words. First of all, there are fewer consonant and vowel sounds in the Spanish language than in English. English sounds such as *th* or *v*, which have no direct counterpart in Spanish, are difficult for many children from Spanish-speaking backgrounds.

Although many consonant sounds are common to both English and Spanish, these consonants are not always produced in exactly the same way in the two languages. The consonant *t*, for example, is aspirated (i.e., followed by a puff of air) in English words, but this same sound is unaspirated in Spanish words. Moreover, the Spanish *t* is dental (i.e., the tongue touches the back of the upper front teeth) while the English *t* is alveolar (i.e., the tongue touches the alveolar ridge above the teeth). Although the differences between English and Spanish productions of the same sounds are often subtle, they contribute to the accent observed when Spanish speakers produce English words.

In contrast to English, where most consonants can occur at the end of words, the only consonants ever *heard* at the end of Spanish words are *n*, *l*, *s*, *r*, and *d*. Thus, Spanish speakers are often observed to produce substitutions or omissions when English words end in sounds other than *n*, *l*, *s*, *r*, or *d*. Substitution of *s* for *z*, for example, would be likely at the end of the word *freeze* (O'Brien, 1973).

A major problem experienced by individuals learning a second language is that they must acquire a whole series of phonemic contrasts that do not exist in their native language. When a language has no phonemic distinctions between two sounds, the speaker of that language may experience difficulty perceiving the two sounds as different (Matluck & Mace, 1973).

Researchers have examined the extent to which errors in the second language can be predicted based on a comparison of linguistic structural differences between the two languages. The viewpoint that errors reflecting the structure of the first language are produced when structures differ in the two languages is called the *contrastive analysis hypothesis* (Anderson, 1981; Dulay, Burt, & Krashen, 1982; Locke, 1981). The analysis of the phonological performance of second language learners, however, has revealed that contrastive analysis cannot account for many of their errors (Dickerson, 1974; Wardhaugh, 1970). Anderson (1981) argued that the contrastive analysis hypothesis is inadequate as an explanation of the phonological errors produced by second language learners:

> The assumption that the native language of the learner is an accurate predictor of second language errors is no longer tenable. The acquisition of the phonology of a second language is far more complex than previously thought; there is no simple formula for predicting the second language learner's errors. (p. 94)

A contrastive analysis of English and Spanish was developed by Stockwell and Bowen (1965) based on the assumption that second language learners would have greatest difficulty with sounds in the second language that are most different from those in the first language. Their proposed hierarchy of difficulty for speech sounds in the second language, however, does not correspond to the order in which speech sounds are actually acquired by second language learners. Based on a review of data reported in several studies, Dulay, Hernandez-Chavez, and Burt (1978) reported that "most of the currently available evidence, meager though it is, suggests strongly that L2 [Language 2] acquisition follows a developmental course that is strikingly similar to that of L1" (pp. 284–285). It appears that sounds acquired late in the developmental sequence by monolingual speakers also tend to be acquired late by second language learners.

Dulay et al. (1982) maintain that the phonological system of the first language is used as a base in the development of a second language phonology. Thus, the child starts with the sounds, sound sequences, and rules of the first language and gradually develops skill in differentiating between the two phonological systems as greater experience is acquired in using the second language. It appears that a developmental process takes place in which the child, over a period of time, comes to acquire the phonological rules necessary for the correct production of speech sounds in the second language. This process shows many similarities to that observed among first language learners.

Second language learners who demonstrate difficulties in the pronunciation of English words should be considered to have articulation disorders only if evidence of delayed phonological development is identified in their first language. If assessment is conducted only in English, it is difficult to distinguish phonological behaviors that are indicative of a disorder from those that reflect normal developmental processes in the acquisition of a second phonology:

> Assessment for the purpose of identifying speech disorders should always be done in the first, or dominant, language of the child. At present, there are no reliable means to determine whether a child's articulation errors in the second language reflect the child's interlanguage phonology or whether they are evidence of a speech disorder. Consequently, testing for articulation disorders in the second language could result in labeling a normal child as handicapped. In addition, a program of speech therapy might interfere with the child's normal interlanguage development. (Anderson, 1981, p. 96)

The phonological differences produced by second language learners are to be expected and must not be viewed as disorders. The developmental processes that occur during the acquisition of a second language phonology must be recognized and understood by assessment personnel so that children are not incorrectly diagnosed as handicapped.

Language Disorders

Language disorders may affect the form, content, or the functional use of language. Because language disorders affect common processes underlying the different surface manifestations of both languages, it is not possible for a bilingual child to have a language disorder in one language and not in the other (Juarez, 1983). Limited English proficient children who are able to communicate normally in their native language do not have language disorders and, therefore, are not appropriate candidates for remedial programs. The following factors should be considered when assessing bilingual children for possible language disorders:

The bilingual child's language performance should be compared to that of other bilingual speakers who have had similar cultural and linguistic experiences. Bilingual children are a heterogeneous group in terms of the extent to which they have been provided with functional opportunities to use their two languages in various settings in the environment. Therefore, patterns of language use in the home, school, and community need to be examined so that assessment data can be interpreted accurately.

Some bilingual children attend schools where they are provided with instruction only in English, whereas others attend schools where bilingual education programs are available. Moreover, the extent to which the native language and English are used in the home environment varies from family to family. It must not be assumed that all bilingual children have had similar language experiences.

We have encountered numerous cases in the schools where English-dominant children from bilingual backgrounds have been misdiagnosed as having language disorders when their performance in English fell below that of monolingual Anglo children. Children from bilingual backgrounds, however, have often had fewer opportunities to hear and use the English language than have children from homes where only English is used. Therefore, it is normal for these second language learners to demonstrate a lower-level of English language proficiency than the typical monolingual English-speaking child.

A child should be considered to have a language disorder only if language behaviors are exhibited that are atypical of peers from the same cultural group who speak the same dialect and who have had similar opportunities to hear and use the language. The child's language background needs to be considered in the interpretation of assessment data.

Grammatical errors in the second language that are similar to those observed among first language learners are to be expected and must not be viewed as evidence of a disorder. The processes involved in the acquisition of grammar in the second language are similar, in many respects, to those involved in first language acquisition (Dulay et al., 1982). Studies have provided evidence that second language learners progress through an ordered series of stages in the acquisition of grammatical structures in the second language. Milon (1974), for example, found that a Japanese child learning English progressed through stages in the acquisition of negation that were similar to those described by Klima and Bellugi (1966) for first language learners. Other investigators, however, have found that second language learners progress through stages in the acquisition of English language structures, but that these stages are not identical to those observed among native English speakers (Cancino, Rosansky, & Schumann, 1978; Ravem, 1968).

Evidence has also been found that second language learners from a variety of language backgrounds acquire groups of language structures in a fairly set order (Dulay & Burt, 1973, 1974, 1975; Fathman, 1975; Makino, 1979). The acquisition order for 13 English grammatical morphemes is described by Dulay et al. (1982). Group I of this hierarchy, the earliest acquired structures, consists of pronoun case and word order in simple declarative sentences; Group II consists of the singular copula (*'s/is*), singular auxiliary (*'s/is*), plural auxiliary (*are*), and the progressive (*-ing*); Group III consists of the past irregular, possessive (*'s*), conditional auxiliary (*would*), long plural (*-es*), and third-person singular (*-s*); Group IV, the grammatical structures acquired last in the sequence, consists of the perfect auxiliary (*have*) and the past participle (*-en*).

Most research studies on acquisition order in the second language have involved the cross-sectional sampling of the language behavior of different age groups rather than the longitudinal analysis of individual children's linguistic development. In a longitudinal study of six Spanish-speaking children, Rosansky (1976) found that the acquisition order for grammatical morphemes obtained using the Bilingual Syntax Measure did not always resemble the order obtained when spontaneous speech samples in the second language were analyzed. Longitudinal studies of second language learner's development of grammatical structures in spontaneous speech are needed before definitive conclusions can be reached about the existence of an invariant acquisition sequence for second language learners.

Few of the grammatical errors produced in the second language can be attributed to the influence of the first language (Dulay & Burt, 1974; Gillis & Weber, 1976; Milon, 1974). Based on the research findings, Dulay et al. (1982) maintained that only 5% of the grammatical errors made by children in the second language and at most 20% of those made by adults reflect the structure of the first language. The majority of grammatical errors produced by second language learners appear to be developmental errors similar to those observed among children learning a first language.

In our experience with second language learners, we have found that errors sometimes occur on grammatical structures in the second language that cause no difficulty for the child in the first language. It is not uncommon, for example, to observe Spanish-speaking children omitting plural endings on

English nouns even though no difficulty is demonstrated on the Spanish plural noun ending. Other researchers have reported similar observations (Hernandez-Chavez, 1972).

We have observed numerous cases where bilingual children demonstrated inappropriate usage of masculine and feminine pronouns in English even though these pronouns were used correctly in Spanish. The following language sample was obtained from a 7-year-old Spanish-speaking male learning English as a second language: "I have one sister. My sister go to school. He like to see cartoons. My sister got a jacket. He got a doll. And my sister is in my class. He's seven." In the language sample the child consistently substituted *he* for *she* when referring to his sister. Similar errors in pronoun production are often observed among first language learners. This child did not have a language disorder. Rather, the errors produced reflected his limited experience in using the English language.

In the assessment of bilingual children, it is necessary to evaluate their progress in acquiring a system of rules for the construction of utterances. It must be recognized that many of the grammatical errors produced in English by second language learners may be similar to those produced by monolingual English speakers with delayed language development. Therefore, it is difficult to identify bilingual children with language disorders accurately if testing is conducted only in English—proficiency in the minority language should also be examined.

Language loss is a normal phenomenon when opportunities to hear and use the first language are withdrawn or minimized. As children acquire proficiency in a second language, an actual loss of proficiency in the first language occurs in many instances:

> Juanita, a Spanish-speaking child with limited proficiency in English was placed in a foster home at 5 years of age. English was the only language spoken by her foster parents. When Juanita entered kindergarten, she was placed in a kindergarten classroom where all instruction was provided in English. Moreover, all of the other children in the classroom were monolingual English speakers. As Juanita became more proficient in English, she began to lose proficiency in Spanish. English soon became her dominant language.

The child described above was living in an environment where opportunities for the functional use of her native language had been withdrawn. Thus, growth in the second language was accompanied by an actual loss of proficiency in the native language.

Limited English proficient children who experience language loss in their native language may demonstrate language test scores similar to those of bilingual children with language disorders. Factors in the environment that may be contributing to the interruption of development in the native language need to be identified. A detailed case history and an analysis of how each language is used in various speaking contexts is necessary so that children experiencing language loss are not incorrectly diagnosed as language disordered.

Shifting from one language to another within utterance is not necessarily an indicator of language confusion or a language disorder. Two phenomena, *linguistic borrowing* (code mixing) and *code switching*, need to be distinguished from one another. The first of these, linguistic borrowing, involves the incorporation of linguistic elements from one language into another. Borrowed words often reflect concepts that may have been first encountered upon contact with individuals from a different culture or language background. A word such as *freeway*, for example, is likely to be used by immigrants to the Western United States who have had no previous experience with freeways in their native country.

The second phenomenon, code switching, involves alternations back and forth between languages and is not limited to single words. Several shifts between languages may be observed within a single sentence. Code switching may occur at the word, phrase, or sentence level. Bilingual speakers do not tend to alternate between languages in a random fashion. Rather, code switching typically occurs at specific syntactic boundaries (e.g., at the beginning of verb phrases) and maintains the internal structural consistency of the utterance (Dulay et al., 1982).

Code switching is common among individuals who have acquired nativelike fluency in two languages and, therefore, should not be viewed as an abnormal behavior. An individual with a language disorder, however, may alternate between languages because of the language deficit:

> Pedro, a Spanish-speaking male with limited English proficiency, demonstrated a moderate receptive and expressive language impairment resulting from damage to the left cerebral hemisphere. During conversation in Spanish, word retrieval problems were frequent, and he often hesitated for long periods of time in an effort to think of an appropriate word. When unable to recall the word, Pedro would sometimes give the English equivalent.
>
> During an interview with family members, it was learned that Pedro rarely used English in the home prior to the onset of the language disorder. Since that time, however, he has been observed to make use of English words in a number of situations when he was unable to recall the appropriate Spanish vocabulary.

The individual described above made use of his second language when he was unable to recall particular words in his native language. Thus, alternations between languages were a reflection of particular problems that the individual was experiencing in using vocabulary.

The code switching behavior commonly observed among normal bilingual speakers allows for greater precision in the expression of culturally related concepts and serves to enhance the effectiveness of the communication.

Because code switching is a normal behavior, children should not be referred for assessment based solely on the fact that they are observed to switch between languages:

> It is very clear that code switching, far from constituting a breakdown of a bilingual's grammatical system or being an uncontrolled and meaningless *Mischsprache*, is a systematic and meaningful mode of communication for many bilingual communities. It is not "interference" or an abnormality in the speech of a person. On the contrary, code alternation represents the creative use of both languages by the bilingual community. As bilinguals learn the usage norms of two languages within the community, they use them to facilitate the total act of communication. (Dulay et al., 1982, p. 118)

CONTEXTUAL FACTORS AND LANGUAGE ASSESSMENT

A comprehensive evaluation of the bilingual child's communication must include the assessment of both language structure and the child's competence in making functional use of the language. The fact that a child performs well on a test designed to assess particular language structures does not necessarily mean that the individual is able to communicate effectively. Thus, one must examine what the child can *do* with language in natural speaking contexts:

> One important fact about speaking and understanding language is that it always takes place in a context. We do not simply "know" our mother tongue as an abstract system of vocal signals, or as if it was some sort of a grammar book with a dictionary attached. We know it in the sense of knowing how to use it; we know how to communicate with other people, how to choose forms of language that are appropriate to the type of situation we find ourselves in, and so on. (Halliday, 1978, p. 13)

The assessment of competence in functional language use requires an examination of the child's ability to communicate in a variety of roles and contexts. When communication is assessed in context, it is possible to consider the various sociocultural factors in the environment that may be influencing the child's linguistic development. Halliday (1978) emphasized that the social structure is responsible for the meanings that an individual will associate with particular social contexts. The form that social relations take influences the kind of choices in meaning that will be given prominence in different types of situations (Halliday, 1978; Hymes, 1974; Mehrabian, 1972).

The specific functions for which language is used and the discourse rules that govern how individuals interact with one another vary from culture to culture (Fishman, 1972). Cultural groups differ, for example, in the rules governing how individuals take turns during conversations (Hall, 1966; McDermott, 1977). The use of nonverbal behaviors such as eye contact, space and interpersonal distance, facial displays, and body movement during communicative interactions also varies across cultures (Adler, 1979; Ekman, 1973; Sommer, 1969). These differences may be inappropriately labeled as abnormalities if assessment personnel fail to consider the sociocultural environment in which the language is used.

The assessment of communication in context provides data that reflect the child's experiences in using the language. This approach allows one to examine the functions that each language serves for the individual and to determine the child's effectiveness in using the language for specific purposes.

CONSIDERATIONS IN TESTING THE HEARING-IMPAIRED

Hearing-impaired children may exhibit abnormalities in all areas of speech and language development. Children with congenital hearing impairments who are classified as *deaf* do not have enough usable hearing to acquire the spoken language naturally in their environment. The speech that they develop through formal programs of instruction generally is characterized by poor articulation, abnormal temporal and intonational patterns, and a voice quality that is breathy and nasalized (Silverman, 1971). Children who are classified as *hard of hearing*, on the other hand, have enough hearing to learn to speak, although specific deficits may be observed (Grant, 1983; West & Ansberry, 1968). A hard of hearing child with a high-frequency loss, for example, may demonstrate articulation errors that are limited to high-frequency sounds such as *s* or *sh*.

Hearing-impaired children from non-English-speaking homes have generally been placed in programs for the hearing impaired where English is the only language of instruction (Grant, 1983). Thus, these children often acquire the ability to communicate orally and/or sign only in English even though a language other than English may be used in the home. Hard of hearing children, however, have enough usable hearing to develop language in their environment and, therefore, acquire some level of proficiency in the home language prior to formal intervention in an instructional setting. This knowledge of a language other than English must be considered in assessment.

When bilingual, hearing-impaired children are assessed, speech and language behaviors that reflect the individual's limited English proficiency must not be confused with problems that are a product of the hearing impairment. Misarticulation of the *sh* sound, for example, is common among Spanish speakers learning English as a second language. This same sound, however, is often misarticulated by native English speakers with high-frequency hearing losses. When testing is conducted only in English, the distinction between differences and disorders is difficult to make. Therefore, procedures are needed so that the child's auditory functioning and communicative functioning can be examined in the native language.

A comprehensive audiological evaluation is an essential first step in the assessment of bilingual, hearing-impaired children with suspected communicative disorders. The information obtained from the audiological testing is helpful in determining the impact of the hearing impairment on the child's ability to comprehend and use the spoken language.

METHODS FOR COLLECTING ASSESSMENT INFORMATION

Assessment data must be obtained that are representative of the child's communicative capabilities. It should never be assumed that data obtained from a single assessment instrument are accurate:

> Once you have gathered some performance data, assume it is wrong. Do not trust the data from single recording sessions or single data points. Always look for confirming data by comparing the results of different procedures, for example, free-speech analysis versus elicited production of Wh-questions. (Miller, 1981, p. 171)

Procedures that can be used to obtain measures of the child's speech and language behavior include standardized tests, nonstandardized instruments, and natural communication samples.

1. ***Standardized tests.*** Standardized tests can be used to assess specific aspects of the spoken language and to compare the child's performance to that of others. These measures have been used in the field of speech–language pathology primarily in the assessment of articulation and language.

It is not always possible to locate a standardized test with norms that are appropriate for the bilingual population being assessed. Children with communicative disorders, however, can be identified without standardized tests if their language behavior is observed systematically and compared to that of peers who have had similar language experiences. One can also examine the extent to which the child has mastered the skills necessary to meet the linguistic demands of the classroom curriculum.

2. ***Nonstandardized instruments.*** Criterion-referenced tests and other informal measures (e.g., observational checklists) can be used to examine the child's performance on specific speech and language behaviors. Informal measures designed to elicit specific communicative behaviors are often helpful when those behaviors do not occur frequently enough for analysis in recorded samples of the child's natural communication.

3. ***Natural communication samples.*** Performance on formal and informal assessment instruments should always be compared to performance during conversational speech. The communication sample is an essential clinical tool in assessment because it represents how the child uses the language in real life situations (Prutting, 1983).

The specific procedures used in assessment depend on the nature of the referral. Assessment personnel must be responsive to individual differences among children if assessment is to be conducted in a nonbiased manner. Use of a "standard assessment battery" with all speakers of a particular language is not recommended because of the heterogeneity of the bilingual student population (Mattes, 1982c). The appropriateness of assessment instruments must be determined for each child based on an examination of that child's cultural and linguistic background. Moreover, a detailed case history and an analysis of language usage patterns in the child's environment are needed so that cultural and environmental influences can be considered in the interpretation of the assessment data.

THE CURRENT DILEMMA

Public Law 94-142 (1975) requires that testing be conducted using procedures that are nondiscriminatory. If bilingual children with suspected communicative disorders are to be assessed in a nonbiased manner, procedures are needed so that testing can be conducted in both languages. The process of assessing a limited English proficient child's oral communication is difficult when there are few bilingual speech–language pathologists available.

The procedures used in the identification of communicatively handicapped Spanish-speaking children were examined by Mattes (1982c). A survey completed by 154 public school speech–language pathologists revealed that the number of speech–language pathologists with sufficient fluency in Spanish to assess Spanish-speaking children was inadequate to meet the local needs. The study also revealed that commercially available language assessment instruments often did not provide sufficient information to identify Spanish-speaking children with language disorders. The use of Spanish-speaking personnel other than speech–language pathologists in test administration was common. As a result of the shortage of bilingual assessment personnel, however, it was not always possible for speech–language pathologists to ensure that Spanish-speaking children were assessed in Spanish.

The problems encountered by speech–language pathologists in the assessment of Spanish-speaking children are likely to be even more difficult to resolve when children need to be tested who speak minority languages that are less common than Spanish. There are currently few language assessment instruments available for speakers of most minority languages. Moreover, there are few individuals available with the language background and training necessary to conduct assessments when children who speak languages such as Tagalog, Samoan, or Navajo need to be tested.

The development and implementation of nonbiased procedures for the assessment of bilingual children require that speech–language pathologists work closely with professionals from a variety of disciplines. By working closely with administrators, special education specialists, bilingual specialists, and others in the school setting, a team approach to assessment can be developed. The use of a team approach facilitates the appropriate referral of bilingual children for testing and should result in improved practices for identifying communicatively handicapped bilingual individuals.

SUMMARY AND CONCLUSION

Many children enter schools in the United States each year speaking a language other than English. Limited English proficient children are at a definite disadvantage if the school curriculum does not provide opportunities for instruction in the native language. Activities designed to teach English as a second language should be provided within the regular education curriculum. Remedial speech–language programs are appropriate only for bilingual children who demonstrate *specific disorders* in the comprehension and/or use of the spoken language. Bilingual children who lack proficiency in English because of limited opportunities to use the language are not handicapped and, therefore, do not need a remedial program.

It must not be assumed that there is a single standard of language performance that can be used to measure the communicative ability of all speakers of a particular language. Bilingual children differ in the extent to which they have been exposed to their native language and English. Moreover, children who speak the same language do not all speak the same dialect. Dialect differences result from differences in the language environment and, therefore, must not be viewed as deficiencies requiring a remedial program.

Nonbiased assessment entails the elimination of barriers to successful performance so that individuals from different cultural and linguistic backgrounds will have equal opportunities for success. Therefore, the procedures used in the collection and interpretation of the speech–language assessment data should be individualized to reflect the experiences of the children being assessed. It is important to examine the child's effectiveness in using language functionally in natural speaking contexts. When the complex pattern of interactions between the child and the language environment is studied, the probability of misdiagnosis is minimized.

Chapter 2

Developing a Bilingual Assessment Team

It is essential that a team approach be used in the speech–language assessment of children from bilingual backgrounds. The team should include the speech–language pathologist and any other individuals who have knowledge and/or skills that might be of value in the assessment process. Educational psychologists, bilingual education specialists, classroom teachers, bilingual community members, and trained instructional aides are among those who might be included as members of the team. The team approach facilitates the integration of linguistic, cultural, and educational information so that an accurate diagnosis of the problem can be made.

The role served by various members of the team in the assessment of bilingual children varies depending on the specific purpose of the testing and the nature of the problem presented by the child. The speech–language pathologist, for example, may need to consult with bilingual education teachers and members of the child's ethnic group to identify specific cultural factors that may have relevance in the interpretation of assessment data. It may be necessary for monolingual speech–language pathologists to obtain assistance from individuals who speak the child's language when assessment needs to be conducted in a language other than English. The assistance of interpreters is necessary when information needs to be conveyed to the child's parents. The task of identifying communicatively handicapped bilingual children is not easy when there are no speech–language pathologists available who are able to communicate fluently in the child's language.

The extent to which speech–language pathologists are able to participate directly in the testing process depends on their level of fluency in the language in which testing is to be conducted and their knowledge of procedures for identifying communicative disorders in bilingual children. Many of the speech–language pathologists working in school settings have had no formal coursework relevant to issues in the speech–language assessment of bilingual students. To serve effectively as a member of the assessment team requires that the speech–language pathologist have an understanding of the processes involved in first and second language acquisition and knowledge of the factors that distinguish communicative differences from communicative disorders. The speech–language pathologist must become familiar with instruments for assessing language dominance and proficiency in bilingual children, procedures for conducting assessments in a nondiscriminatory manner, and methods for analyzing the effect of cultural and environmental influences on language behavior.

Comprehensive programs of in-service training are necessary if speech–language pathologists are to serve effectively in developing and implementing procedures for assessing the communicative capabilities of bilingual children. School districts should work closely with community organizations and with institutions of higher learning so that comprehensive training programs can be provided for practicing speech–language pathologists. Local needs must be identified so that appropriate training programs can be planned.

The actual testing of children in languages other than English cannot be conducted by a monolingual speech–language pathologist. If a comprehensive program of in-service education is provided, however, both monolingual and bilingual speech–language pathologists can serve important functions in the development of a bilingual assessment team and in coordinating the activities of individual team members. Specific responsibilities of the speech–language pathologist include the following:

The speech–language pathologist should participate in the development of strategies for the collection of the assessment data. The speech–language pathologist is responsible for ensuring that appropriate assessment instruments are used, that the testing is conducted in a nondiscriminatory manner, and that all assessment procedures mandated by PL 94-142 (1975) are implemented. Strategies for collecting natural communication samples, analyzing language usage patterns, and so forth, can be designed by the speech–language pathologist.

The speech–language pathologist should participate in the development of procedures for selecting and training personnel who will participate in various aspects of the assessment process. It is the speech–language pathologist's responsibility to ensure that the individuals involved in test administration have been trained for their roles. Therefore, the speech–language pathologist should be responsible for determining the specific competencies that assessment personnel must have and the specific procedures that will be used to provide them with these competencies.

In addition to their role in test administration, team members can serve as referral sources and interpreters. Training programs need to be developed by the speech–language pathologist so that team members can serve effectively in these roles.

The speech–language pathologist should participate in the review of all speech–language assessment data and in educational decision making. The monolingual speech–language pathologist cannot determine whether a bilingual child has a communicative disorder without assistance from members of the assessment team. The speech–language pathologist's task is to ask questions and to determine if sufficient information has been obtained to indicate the nature of the child's problem. The identification of children with handicaps requires that a *team decision* be reached.

Administrators in school settings must realize that there simply are not enough bilingual speech–language pathologists to meet the needs of the bilingual student population. The development of programs for training personnel to serve as members of a bilingual assessment team is necessary if bilingual children with communicative disorders and other handicaps are to be identified and served appropriately.

PLANNING FOR CHANGE IN ASSESSMENT PRACTICES

School personnel often find themselves faced with a crisis when a bilingual child is referred for testing and there are no assessment personnel available who speak the child's language. The population of bilingual children in our schools is growing and, undoubtedly, will continue to grow. If the needs of these children are to be met, changes will be required in the traditional roles of speech–language pathologists and other professionals in the educational system. School districts must become involved in the development of strategies so that testing can be conducted in languages other than English.

Conducting a Needs Assessment

The change process should begin with an analysis of current problems. By conducting a *needs assessment,* it is possible to identify the type, depth, and scope of problems that have been experienced within the school district in the speech–language assessment of bilingual children. The results of the needs assessment can be useful in planning more effective assessment strategies and in identifying specific areas in which staff development programs are needed.

Kaufman (1972) described needs assessment as a discrepancy analysis—the identification and documentation of differences between the current condition and the desired condition. A comprehensive needs assessment includes all elements of the context in which change is to occur. Examples of some of the questions that should be examined are the following:

1. What procedures are being used to identify those bilingual children who should be referred for speech–language evaluations?
2. To what extent have previous referrals been appropriate?
3. To what extent has testing been conducted in languages other than English when limited English proficient children have been referred for assessment?
4. What personnel and test instruments have been used to test children in languages other than English?
5. How have speech–language pathologists and other school personnel been trained for their roles in the speech–language assessment of bilingual children?

6. What methods have been used to interpret the results of assessment instruments administered in languages other than English?
7. What specific problems have been experienced in the use of test instruments and personnel when bilingual children were assessed?

It is also important to examine the composition of the bilingual student population within the school district and to consider how this population has changed over time. If the Vietnamese student population has tripled during the past year and is expected to continue to increase, the school district should take immediate action to develop strategies for assessing children from this group.

A variety of methods can be used to identify the type, depth, and scope of the problems being experienced by a school district in the assessment of bilingual children. Three suggested approaches are (1) the review of school records, (2) direct observation of assessment practices, and (3) the use of interview techniques and/or questionnaires to obtain information from school personnel.

Review of School Records

A review of student referral forms for speech–language evaluations, test protocols, transcribed communication samples, narrative reports, and other records available within the school setting can reveal specific problems encountered in the assessment process. Records of student referrals make it possible to compare the referral rate for limited English proficient students to that for monolingual English-speaking students. Information reported on referral forms is helpful in assessing the extent to which previous referrals have been appropriate.

Test information contained within individual students' files can be examined to identify the specific procedures that have been used to identify children with communicative disorders. If the assessment battery used to assess limited English proficient children is found to consist entirely of tests administered in English, one needs to find out why testing has not been conducted in the child's first language.

Direct Observation

Observational techniques can be used to study the actual delivery of assessment services to bilingual children. A consultant with expertise in the assessment of bilingual children, for example, could be asked to observe local school personnel administer tests to bilingual children. Based on the observations, the consultant may be able to identify specific areas in which staff development programs are needed.

Interviews and Questionnaires

Interview techniques and questionnaires can be used to identify the specific concerns of speech–language pathologists, teachers, administrators, and others in the school setting. Data reflecting their understanding of the assessment process and their perceived needs must be obtained so that specific areas can be identified in which changes should be implemented.

Use of the Needs Assessment Data

The results of the needs assessment should be reviewed by a team of professionals. Thus, speech–language pathologists should work closely with school administrators, bilingual specialists, and other school personnel in the development of solution strategies for the specific problems identified.

Changes in assessment practices are not likely to occur without support from the school administration. It is essential that the results of the needs assessment be shared with school administrators from both regular and special education. School principals often can suggest procedures for using bilingual school personnel (e.g., bilingual paraprofessionals) in the assessment process. The special education coordinator may be willing to make contacts with other school districts and various agencies in the community in an effort to locate bilingual professionals with expertise in speech–language assessment.

Based on the information obtained from the needs assessment, existing problems can be identified and plans can be developed for a specific course of action. Close cooperation among team members is essential if assessment procedures are to be developed that adequately meet the needs of the local bilingual student population.

REFERRAL AND ASSESSMENT: A TEAM APPROACH

A total program of staff development is necessary if a team approach is to be implemented effectively within the school setting. In-service education should be provided for school administrators to sensitize them to the problems that often are encountered in efforts to use tests and assessment personnel in a nondiscriminatory manner. Classroom teachers and other school personnel must be provided with in-service education so that they can identify bilingual children who should be referred to the speech–language pathologist. Individuals who participate directly in test administration need to be trained to administer tests. Finally, programs are needed to provide team members with the skills necessary to coordinate their efforts both in data collection and in the interpretation of the test results.

An important first step in the training of school personnel is to provide these individuals with general information about the assessment process and the complex issues involved in identifying communicatively handicapped bilingual children. Topics that should be included in these in-service programs include the following:

1. Current laws and their relevance in the speech–language assessment of bilingual children;
2. Rationale for using a team approach in assessment;

3. Factors to consider in distinguishing between normal and abnormal speech–language development when observing bilingual children;
4. Procedures for implementing classroom screening programs;
5. Procedures for making speech–language referrals;
6. Criteria for enrolling bilingual children in speech–language remediation.

The Referral Process

Referrals for speech–language evaluations generally come from classroom instructional personnel, school nurses, and others within the school setting who have direct contact with students. A teacher who refers every bilingual student in the classroom to the speech–language pathologist probably is making referrals that are not appropriate. Similarly, a teacher who is hesitant to refer bilingual children for testing may be overlooking true disorders.

The speech–language pathologist must provide school personnel with sufficient information about communicative disorders and bilingualism so that they can make appropriate referrals. School personnel must understand that bilingual children do not have communicative disorders if their observed difficulties in using language are limited to the second language. An example of an inappropriate referral follows:

> Pierre was referred to the speech–language pathologist on the first day of school by his classroom teacher. The child was born in France and speaks French fluently and without difficulty. He has only been in the United States for 2 weeks.
>
> The referral form submitted to the speech–language pathologist by the classroom teacher contained the following information: "Pierre is the only French-speaking child in my classroom. I feel that he should be seen by the speech pathologist for English language instruction."

The child described above was referred to the speech–language pathologist for testing because he did not speak English. Rather than speech–language remediation, this child needs a modified regular education curriculum designed to meet the needs of a non-English speaker.

Classroom teachers sometimes seek assistance from speech–language pathologists when difficulties are encountered in providing limited English proficient children with appropriate programs of second language instruction. It is recommended that speech–language pathologists serve in a *consulting* role when teachers need assistance in teaching English to nonhandicapped second-language learners. The speech–language pathologist, for example, could demonstrate specific instructional techniques and provide teachers with guidance as these techniques are implemented in the regular classroom. Enrollment in a program for individuals with communicative disorders, however, is appropriate only for those bilingual children who demonstrate evidence of specific abnormalities in their acquisition of language.

Classroom teachers may, on occasion, refer limited English proficient children for testing who appear to be having more difficulty acquiring English than other children in the classroom. The fact that a child is learning English more slowly than peers is a valid reason for concern and may reflect an underlying language disorder in some cases. Langdon (1983) found that a group of 25 Spanish-speaking children judged by their teachers to be progressing normally in their development of English performed better on tasks in both English and Spanish than a group of 25 Spanish-speaking children judged by their teachers "as having difficulty comprehending and/or expressing English when compared to other children of similar backgrounds" (p. 42). Thus, the possibility that a communicative disorder is present should be considered when a teacher expresses concern that a child is acquiring English at a much slower rate than other second language learners in the classroom. The administration of a classroom screening measure in the child's native language is recommended to determine if the child is also experiencing difficulty communicating in that language. If problems are evident in the native language also, the child should be referred for a formal speech–language evaluation.

Classroom Screening Procedures

Monolingual classroom teachers have difficulty identifying limited English proficient children who should be referred for speech–language evaluations without assistance from individuals who are bilingual. Therefore, an important function of the assessment team is to develop screening procedures that can be implemented within the regular classroom setting by bilingual individuals (e.g., bilingual paraprofessionals) who have been trained specifically to conduct the screening.

The use of structured articulation and language screening tests to identify possible candidates for remedial speech–language programs has been popular in public school settings. When administered to bilingual children, only those individuals who demonstrate evidence of communication problems in *both* languages should be referred to the speech–language pathologist for further testing.

In schools where language dominance tests are administered to bilingual children, it may be possible to coordinate the speech–language screening procedures with the language dominance testing. Thus, personnel involved in the administration of language dominance tests could be trained to record specific communication problems that were observed during the testing.

A major problem with structured screening tests is that they typically focus on specific structural features of the language rather than on the child's pragmatic communication capabilities. Pragmatic measures, however, have been found to be better predictors of academically consequential language disorders in bilingual populations (Damico, Oller, & Storey, 1983).

Screening can also be conducted by having bilingual speakers systematically observe children's communicative interactions with peers who speak the same language. Their observations can be recorded on a screening inventory, as shown in the following example:

Child: Refugio Ramos
Language spoken: Spanish

	Communicative behavior	Problem	No problem
1.	Articulates speech sounds correctly.		X
2.	Uses correct grammar.	X	
3.	Uses voice appropriately.		X
4.	Describes experiences accurately.	X	
5.	Uses vocabulary effectively to express ideas.	X	
6.	Sequences statements appropriately.	X	
7.	Maintains topic of discussion.	X	
8.	Follows teacher's instructions.		X
9.	Responds appropriately to questions.	X	
10.	Speaks without excessive pauses, repetitions, false starts, etc.	X	

An example of a more comprehensive inventory is presented in chapter 6. When screening inventories are used, it is possible to record observations of the child's performance in both the structural and functional aspects of communication as language is used in context. The development of classroom screening programs in which bilingual personnel use these inventories should result in more appropriate referrals for speech–language evaluations.

The Assessment Process

The assessment of bilingual children is most difficult when there are no bilingual assessment personnel available locally who can conduct the speech–language testing. When faced with such a situation, it is necessary to make contacts with other resources in an effort to locate bilingual personnel with training and experience in the assessment of bilingual children. Examples of contacts that may be helpful in locating speakers of the child's language are the following:

1. Contacts with other school districts. Other school districts in the community may be able to recommend individuals who have participated in the assessment of bilingual children.

2. Contacts with county/state departments of education. Listings of bilingual specialists can sometimes be obtained from the county or from the state department of education.

3. Contacts with associations such as the American Speech–Language–Hearing Association. The American Speech–Language–Hearing Association currently publishes a Directory of Bilingual Speech–Language Pathologists and Audiologists. The 1982–1983 edition of the directory provides a listing of all members of the Association who have identified themselves as having foreign language skills. A total of 34 languages are represented. The individual listings include the following information: name, highest academic degree, address, phone number, level of proficiency in the language, special skills, and area of clinical certification.

4. Contacts with local colleges and universities. Professors in fields such as speech–language pathology, linguistics, and special education may be able to assist in locating bilingual individuals with competencies in assessment. Foreign language departments may have professors on staff who speak the child's language. Individuals with previous experience in examining children's oral communication are preferred.

5. Contacts with agencies that serve the needs of individuals from minority backgrounds. Agencies that are directly involved in minority concerns (e.g., Lau Centers) may be able to provide information that is helpful in locating bilingual assessment personnel.

6. Contacts with organizations that include individuals from the child's ethnic group. Individuals who speak the child's language can often be located by contacting the church and/or other community organizations attended by the child's family.

When a bilingual speech–language pathologist cannot be located, it becomes necessary to train other personnel for roles in assessment and for roles as interpreters. Bilingual graduate students in speech–language pathology, various professionals in special education and bilingual education, and classroom instructional aides are among the individuals who can be included as members of the assessment team.

Graduate Students in Speech–Language Pathology

Bilingual graduate students in speech–language pathology with clinical experience in the assessment of bilingual children can be a valuable resource when children need to be tested. These individuals can be used both as test administrators and as interpreters. In the absence of a bilingual speech–language pathologist, graduate students in speech–language pathology are often the best qualified individuals available for specific roles in the speech–language assessment of bilingual children.

Professionals in Special Education and Bilingual Education

Bilingual special education specialists (e.g., school psychologists), teachers in bilingual education programs, and other professionals in the school setting who have had previous training and experience in test administration procedures can be considered for roles in assessment. Bilingual education teachers, for example, have often had experience in the actual use of language assessment instruments.

Professional Interpreters

Professional interpreters can be used when information needs to be explained to the child's parents. They also may be able to assist in test administration and test construction. These individuals, however, often do not have the background in special education necessary to serve effectively as interpreters when test results, criteria for special education placement, and other complex educational concepts need to be explained to the parents. Moreover, these individuals are not necessarily familiar with the local dialect or with test administration procedures.

Classroom Instructional Aides and Other Supportive Personnel

Bilingual classroom instructional aides, parent volunteers, and other paraprofessionals may be able to participate in various aspects of the assessment process. These individuals often live in the community and speak the local dialect. Paraprofessionals, however, often have had no experience in giving tests and may not understand the purpose of testing. When efforts to locate bilingual professionals are unsuccessful, however, the use of paraprofessionals may be the only alternative.

Speech–language pathologists must recognize the many problems that can occur when speech–language evaluations are conducted by an individual who is not specifically trained in the field of speech–language pathology. The diagnosis of communicative disorders is especially difficult when a child speaks two languages. Speech–language pathologists cannot afford to risk the possibility that a child is misdiagnosed or that incorrect information is conveyed to the parents about the purpose of the evaluation or the test results. Therefore, care must be taken in the selection, training, and use of all bilingual personnel who participate in various aspects of the assessment process.

Bilingual individuals who have had experience in test administration can provide valuable assistance to monolingual speech–language pathologists in developing and implementing training programs. Classroom instructional aides and other paraprofessionals selected for roles in assessment *must* be trained for all of the specific activities that they will be asked to perform (see chapter 3).

Review of the Assessment Data

It is necessary for the monolingual speech–language pathologist to obtain information from members of the assessment team so that the child's specific needs can be identified—A team approach in decision making is needed. Whenever a bilingual child is assessed by someone other than a bilingual speech–language pathologist, the child's responses should be audiotaped or videotaped so that they can be examined by individual members of the assessment team. It is recommended that the speech–language pathologist discuss the contents of the tape with a minimum of two fluent speakers of the local dialect. These individuals should be interviewed independently so that their observations can be compared. The child's utterances during natural communication activities, responses produced on standardized tests, and so forth, should be discussed. If the reviewers are not in agreement about the specific problems that the child is experiencing, then additional assistance will be needed in the review of the assessment data.

When a child demonstrates a severe communicative disorder, the assessment team is likely to experience little difficulty in determining that the child has special needs. A kindergarten child who is speaking in one-word utterances both at school and at home obviously has a problem. When the problem is more subtle, however, the local review of the child's performance may raise questions that can only be answered by individuals who have expertise in the communicative assessment of bilingual children.

What needs to be determined by the assessment team is whether or not the child demonstrates communicative behaviors that are atypical of peers who have had similar cultural and linguistic experiences. In addition to reviewing the results of testing, the influence of various cultural and environmental factors needs to be examined. If deficits noted in the child's first language reflect language loss that has occurred as a result of limited functional opportunities to use that language, then it would be inappropriate for the assessment team to conclude that the child has a disorder. Thus, the assessment team must consider the child's language history and how each language is used in various contexts when interpreting the assessment findings. General factors that need to be considered in identifying children with communicative disorders are summarized in Table 1.

Following the review of the assessment data at the local level, the speech–language pathologist may still have questions that need to be answered before an educational decision can be reached. It may be possible to send test information and audiotaped or videotaped samples of the child's communication to a bilingual speech–language pathologist for further analysis when there are no bilingual speech–language pathologists available locally. Care must be taken, however, in selecting a speech–language pathologist who has the skills necessary to conduct the analysis. If a directory of bilingual speech–language pathologists is used, for example, it is important to consider level of language proficiency, training, and experience prior to selecting anyone to assist in reviewing the test results.

Glass (1979) suggested that an international registry and language bank be established to assist speech–language pathologists in the assessment of bilingual individuals. The speech–language pathologist could then provide the language bank with audiotapes or videotapes of the child's performance,

TABLE 1.
Considerations in Reviewing Limited English Proficient Children's Language Assessment Results

Results of testing	Diagnosis	Action
Problems noted only in English.	Not a communicative disorder.	Child does not qualify for a remedial speech–language program. Consultation with bilingual education personnel is suggested to develop a culturally and linguistically appropriate program within the regular education curriculum.
Problems noted in both languages. Language loss is responsible for the deficits observed in the first language.	Not a communicative disorder. Language loss in the first language is a normal phenomenon when functional opportunities to use the first language are withdrawn or minimized.	Child does not qualify for a remedial speech–language program. Consultation with bilingual education personnel is suggested to develop an appropriate regular education curriculum for the child.
Problems noted in both languages. Language loss is not a factor.	Possible communicative disorder if the problems noted cannot be accounted for by differences in dialect, cultural background, etc. The extent to which the child has had functional opportunities to use each language should be considered.	Child qualifies for a remedial speech–language program if communicative behaviors are identified that are atypical of other children who have had similar cultural and linguistic experiences. Placement in speech–language remediation is appropriate only if the child's needs cannot be met within the regular classroom.

a detailed case report, and other relevant information. A group of bilingual speech–language pathologists might participate in the analysis of the information submitted. To be successful in accurately identifying communicative disorders, however, the speech–language pathologists reviewing the data would have to be familiar with the child's dialect and with the complex environmental variables that may be having an impact on the child's performance. Thus, this approach can be successful only if the speech–language pathologists participating in data analysis are able to discuss the case with assessment personnel at the child's school and with the child's parents.

The extent to which local bilingual assessment teams are able to interpret assessment findings without outside assistance depends on the competencies of individual team members and the specific nature of the problem demonstrated by the child. Sometimes the child's problem is obvious. Other cases, however, may require expertise that is not available locally. Therefore, speech–language pathologists should seek assistance from outside resources when problems are experienced by the local bilingual assessment team in the analysis or interpretation of the assessment data.

NEED FOR BILINGUAL SPEECH–LANGUAGE PROGRAM SPECIALISTS

The task of developing effective assessment strategies for bilingual children can be facilitated by hiring bilingual speech–language pathologists specifically for positions as *bilingual speech–language program specialists.* These individuals could provide assistance to school districts in both assessment and program planning. Their roles in assessment should include the following:

1. To assist school districts in selecting and training personnel for roles on the bilingual assessment team;
2. To provide school districts with strategies for using a team approach to conduct assessments in a nondiscriminatory manner;
3. To provide consulting services to school districts when problems are experienced in the delivery of assessment services and/or in the interpretation of assessment findings;
4. To assist school districts in selecting and/or constructing test instruments that are appropriate for use in assessing children from the local population;
5. To participate directly in testing bilingual children when school districts do not have access to bilingual personnel who can conduct the testing;
6. To provide ongoing programs of in-service education to speech–language pathologists, classroom teachers, and other individuals who serve in various roles on the local assessment team.

In addition to having competencies in bilingual assessment procedures, individuals serving as bilingual speech–language program specialists need to have the leadership capabilities necessary to work effectively with school districts in their efforts to improve assessment practices. To serve effectively in a leadership role requires the ability to adapt one's behavior to meet the needs of the group and of the environment in which change is to occur (Hersey & Blanchard, 1977). Therefore, the bilingual speech–language program specialist must be sensitive to the needs of individual school districts so that strategies for change can be planned and implemented effectively.

ESTABLISHING CHANNELS OF COMMUNICATION

Channels of communication need to be established between school districts to facilitate the location and effective use of bilingual speech–language pathologists and other trained bilingual assessment personnel. School districts that have bilingual speech–language pathologists and other bilingual assessment personnel may be able to share these resources with other school districts. The development and distribution of a directory listing bilingual assessment personnel in the local area should be beneficial to school districts when assistance is needed in the assessment of bilingual children.

School districts must work together in the development of programs designed to provide speech–language pathologists and other school personnel with training so that these individuals can serve effectively as members of the bilingual assessment team. School personnel need to have an understanding of bilingualism and the complex problems involved in distinguishing communicative differences from communicative disorders if a bilingual team approach is to be developed and implemented effectively in the school setting.

Chapter 3

Roles for Paraprofessionals in Assessment

Professional recognition of the value of using bilingual paraprofessionals who have been trained specifically for roles in assessment is essential so that school systems can develop more appropriate educational services for children from bilingual backgrounds. The term *bilingual paraprofessional,* as used in this chapter, refers to an individual who assists the speech–language pathologist, classroom teacher, and/or other *professionals* by serving in a supportive role (e.g., classroom instructional aide). The use of bilingual paraprofessionals in the speech–language assessment of bilingual children is sometimes the *only* alternative when there are no bilingual speech–language pathologists available to conduct the testing. A survey completed by 154 public school speech–language pathologists in Los Angeles County, an area with a large Hispanic population, revealed that less than 12% of the respondents spoke Spanish with sufficient fluency to transcribe and analyze samples of conversational speech. The majority of speech–language pathologists working at schools where evaluations had been conducted in Spanish reported that they had made use of assessment personnel other than speech–language pathologists in test administration. Those used most often were bilingual instructional aides (Mattes, 1982c).

The use of paraprofessionals in the field of special education has increased dramatically in recent years (Frith & Teller, 1982; Pickett, 1979). In the field of speech–language pathology, research has provided evidence that paraprofessionals can be effective in providing direct services to children (Carrier, 1970; Costello & Bosler, 1976; Costello & Schoen, 1978; Harris, 1975). Paraprofessionals have provided assistance to speech–language pathologists in assessment, remediation, working with families, clerical activities and in other roles (Alpiner, Ogden & Wiggens, 1970; Mattes, 1982c; Scalero & Eskenazi, 1976). When paraprofessionals are used, it is possible for speech–language pathologists to meet the needs of a larger population of handicapped children.

USING PARAPROFESSIONALS IN A SUPPORTIVE ROLE

Many practicing professionals have serious concerns that bilingual children will be misdiagnosed if speech–language assessment instruments are administered by someone other than a speech–language pathologist. Misdiagnosis is likely to occur if bilingual individuals are asked to participate in testing without first being trained for their roles. The individuals selected may have minimal knowledge of the purpose of the evaluation. Moreover, the speech–language pathologist may have no way of judging their level of proficiency in the language in which the assessment is being conducted (Anderson, 1983).

Whenever a bilingual child is referred for assessment, testing should be conducted, if at all possible, by a bilingual speech–language pathologist. The use of bilingual classroom instructional aides and other paraprofessionals in assessment roles should be considered only in situations where the availability of bilingual speech–language pathologists and other bilingual professionals with experience in testing is insufficient to meet the local demand. The paraprofessionals' limited background in the field of speech–language pathology must be recognized and they must never be used in roles for which they have not been trained. A bilingual paraprofessional who has been trained only to administer screening tests should not be analyzing language samples or serving as an interpreter. The paraprofessional is not a speech–language pathologist and, therefore, must be used only in a supportive role:

> A paraprofessional's primary purpose is to assist the teacher or therapist. Being a successful paraprofessional means willingly accepting a secondary role and implementing directives of the appropriate supervisor. Paraprofessionals should not be viewed as major decision- or policy-makers. To minimize misunderstandings, their relative position in the schools' line-staff personnel chart and their job description should be well defined. (Frith & Teller, 1982, p. 173)

ETHICAL RESPONSIBILITIES OF SPEECH–LANGUAGE PATHOLOGISTS

Bilingual paraprofessionals need to be given training, guidance, and supervision for the roles that they are asked to perform. Speech–language pathologists must have an understanding of their ethical responsibilities in the use of paraprofessionals.

1. The speech–language pathologist should assign paraprofessionals to engage only in those activities for which training has been provided.
2. The speech–language pathologist must develop procedures for supervising paraprofessionals in all of their activities.
3. The speech–language pathologist is responsible for determining which children will be assessed by the paraprofessional and the specific procedures that will be used in the testing.

4. The speech–language pathologist should not assign the responsibility for educational decision making to the paraprofessional. Paraprofessionals should share their observations of specific speech and/or language problems exhibited by the child during testing but should not be responsible for determining how the child's needs will be met. It is the responsibility of the speech–language pathologist to review the test results with all members of the assessment team so that a team decision can be reached.

The Code of Ethics of the American Speech–Language–Hearing Association specifies that speech–language pathologists must assume full responsibility for supportive personnel who are used to offer clinical services. Thus, speech–language pathologists must recognize their role in the development of procedures to ensure that paraprofessionals maintain a high level of competence in their assigned duties.

What needs to be stressed is that *para-* means working *beside* or *together with* the professional. The speech–language pathologist is the one who must assume responsibility for all decisions made during the course of the assessment process.

PROBLEMS IN USING MONOLINGUAL SPEECH–LANGUAGE PATHOLOGISTS AS TRAINERS

It has been our observation that bilingual paraprofessionals often have been trained for assessment roles by speech–language pathologists who do not speak the language in which testing is to be conducted. The following case study illustrates a situation in which this occurred:

> Mack was referred for a special education evaluation by his stepfather on the first day of kindergarten. The child, a 5-year-old male, was born in Japan and had been diagnosed as autistic in that country at 2 years of age. Mack came to the United States at age 4, following his mother's marriage to an American marine. Both English and Japanese were spoken at home with the child.
>
> The speech–language pathologist worked with a bilingual, Japanese-speaking instructional aide and the child's parents to construct basic vocabulary measures in English and Japanese. Receptive vocabulary was assessed using a task in which the child was asked to point to objects named by the examiner while expressive vocabulary was assessed by having the child name objects. The speech–language pathologist demonstrated the administration of the tasks prior to having the instructional aide test the child. The speech–language pathologist also demonstrated techniques for eliciting language samples. Language samples were obtained during play activities at school and in the child's home.

> All assessment data were audiotaped. The content of the tape was reviewed response by response with the instructional aide. The tape was also played for the child's parents and reviewed. Based on this review, it was determined that the child had limited vocabulary in both languages, did not combine words, generally did not respond to verbal stimuli, demonstrated an unusual rise in pitch at the end of words, produced frequent echolalic responses, and made minimal use of either language for communication purposes. From the results of the testing and a detailed case history, it was determined that the child had a severe communicative disorder.

In the above case study, the speech–language pathologist had little difficulty training and using a paraprofessional effectively to identify the child's disorder. This child, however, had a severe disorder that could be identified quite easily in natural speaking situations and on basic vocabulary tasks that required minimal training to administer. The process of training paraprofessionals to obtain sufficient information for the identification of communicative disorders is more difficult when the child's problem is less obvious.

To evaluate a paraprofessional's ability to administer and score an assessment instrument correctly, one must be able to determine what is being said by the examiner and how it is being said. The child's verbal responses and behavior during the testing also need to be examined to determine the paraprofessional's competencies in recording assessment data. Without knowledge of the child's language, for example, the speech–language pathologist would not be able to determine if the paraprofessional is speaking at an appropriate rate, pronouncing words clearly, or recording the child's responses correctly during the administration of an articulation test.

The procedures for administering tests generally are not difficult to explain to a paraprofessional if the speech–language pathologist is familiar with the test manual. Some paraprofessionals, however, may feel uncomfortable asking questions when something is not understood. Other paraprofessionals, however, may not ask questions because it is culturally inappropriate to indicate that material taught was not learned.

Thus, numerous problems can result when a monolingual speech–language pathologist attempts to train bilingual paraprofessionals for roles in assessment. The Code of Ethics of the American Speech–Language–Hearing Association specifies that professional practitioners must not permit services to be provided by others who are not properly prepared to provide these services. Monolingual speech–language pathologists should, if at all possible, work as a member of a *team* in developing and providing training programs for bilingual paraprofessionals. By including fluent bilingual speakers on this team, strategies can be developed that provide paraprofessionals with the competencies necessary to perform their assigned duties.

TRAINING PARAPROFESSIONALS USING A TEAM APPROACH

Training programs for paraprofessionals are most cost effective if school districts in the local community work together to develop strategies for providing the training. When a team approach is used in training paraprofessionals, a bilingual individual with experience in test administration procedures assists monolingual speech–language pathologists in the training process. A bilingual speech–language pathologist, for example, might be hired specifically to work with monolingual speech–language pathologists in providing the training. When assistance cannot be obtained from a speech–language pathologist who has experience in testing bilingual children and the language fluency necessary to conduct the training, other bilingual individuals with training and experience in test administration need to be included on the training team. It is recommended that the training team include a minimum of two bilingual individuals with experience in testing. Bilingual members of the training team, for example, might include a bilingual psychologist who has administered standardized tests to bilingual children, a classroom instructional aide with training and experience in language dominance testing, and a bilingual education teacher who has used criterion-referenced language tests in the classroom setting. By combining their efforts and sharing responsibilities, team members should be able to train paraprofessionals for a variety of assessment roles. Moreover, paraprofessionals who have been trained and used effectively often can provide assistance to speech–language pathologists when additional paraprofessionals need to be trained.

Content of the Training Program

The content of training programs varies depending on local needs and the qualifications of individual members of the training team. A comprehensive program designed to train paraprofessionals for a variety of roles in the assessment process needs to include the following areas:

1. Characteristics of articulation, language, voice, and fluency disorders;
2. Information about first language acquisition, second language acquisition, and problems in distinguishing communicative differences from communicative disorders;
3. Terminology in speech–language pathology and special education that needs to be understood by paraprofessionals who will be asked to explain forms, testing procedures, test results, and so forth, to the parents;
4. Role of the paraprofessional as a member of the assessment team;
5. Goals of speech–language screening and diagnostic testing;
6. Procedures for administering, scoring, and interpreting the specific assessment instruments that will be used by the paraprofessional;
7. Differences in the structure of English and the structure of the language in which testing is to be conducted;

8. Cultural differences that are important to consider in administering tests and in interpreting test results;
9. Working effectively with parents of the children being assessed;
10. Use of the assessment results in educational decision making and program planning;
11. Professional ethics and current laws with special reference to issues in the speech–language assessment of bilingual children.

The extent to which individual paraprofessionals need to participate in training programs in the areas listed above varies depending on their background and the specific assessment role in which they are asked to function. An individual who participates only in the administration of a classroom speech–language screening test, for example, requires a different type of training program from an individual who serves both in test administration and as an interpreter. Thus, the content of the training programs must be tailored to meet the individual needs of the paraprofessionals being trained.

Selection of Paraprofessionals for Training

Prior to selecting paraprofessionals for training, it is important to obtain information about their level of language proficiency, educational background, and experience in working with children. Recommended guidelines for the selection of paraprofessionals are the following:

Paraprofessionals must have the oral language fluency necessary to serve effectively in assessment roles. Each paraprofessional should be interviewed in the language in which assessment duties are to be performed. Individuals who are not able to converse fluently in that language should not be considered for roles in assessment.

Paraprofessionals must have the reading and writing skills necessary to administer tests correctly and to record responses appropriately. The local development of an examination is recommended to assess the individual's ability to read test stimuli orally and to write down information as it is dictated in the native language.

Paraprofessionals must have the ability to relate to children from the particular cultural group that they will be working with in assessment. It is recommended that paraprofessionals be selected who have had previous experience in working with children in school settings and who have references from individuals qualified to verify their capabilities.

Paraprofessionals must be selected who will be able to maintain the confidentiality of school records and who will respect the rights of the child's parents. Paraprofessionals should be selected who will not "tell tales out of school." Paraprofessionals also must not try to influence decisions that are to be made by the child's parents. It is the school's responsibility to select paraprofessionals who will abide by school rules and who can be trusted.

Using Paraprofessionals in Test Administration

Many paraprofessionals in school settings work in an instructional environment in which they have had little opportunity to administer tests to the children. In such an environment, these paraprofessionals are concerned about helping children succeed with their lessons, showing them what to do, and providing assistance whenever difficulties are experienced. Correct answers are praised in this process and wrong answers are corrected. When children make mistakes, they are often given a second chance so that maximum learning will occur.

In a testing situation, however, children are not to be helped when they do not know the answer. There may be several sample items but, for the most part, children must respond on their own. When administering tests, paraprofessionals must understand that clues are not to be provided and that the child is not to be corrected. This can be difficult for paraprofessionals who have worked with children only in an instructional environment.

An additional problem in the testing situation might be labeled "cultural protection." After working for months or years with children from their own culture, paraprofessionals can become quite protective and may feel uncomfortable when these children do not experience success. This reaction may reflect a desire to "save face" for the children or may reflect empathy for other problems that these children have experienced. These barriers may appear even when a child is referred for testing by the paraprofessional.

Direct instruction must be provided in the use of each of the assessment instruments that the paraprofessional is expected to administer in testing children. The purpose of each instrument should be explained and the administration of the instrument should be demonstrated. The training program must also provide paraprofessionals with experience in the administration of each instrument in situations where they are supervised by members of the training team. The bilingual members of the training team have important responsibilities in demonstrating test administration procedures, observing paraprofessionals as they administer tests, and providing monolingual speech–language pathologists with feedback on the performance of the paraprofessionals. By using a team approach in training paraprofessionals, these individuals can acquire the skills necessary to assist speech–language pathologists in test administration and in the collection of language samples.

In addition to using trained bilingual paraprofessionals in test administration when children are referred for evaluations, these individuals can participate in classroom screening programs. Their involvement in classroom screening activities may facilitate the early identification of children with communicative disorders.

Paraprofessionals as Referral Sources

Bilingual paraprofessionals can serve an important function in referring children to the speech–language pathologist who are in need of speech–language remediation. Most paraprofessionals working in school settings, however, have not been provided with training to help them identify children with possible communicative disorders. When assisting the classroom teacher in providing language and reading instruction to limited English proficient children, the paraprofessional may experience distress or dismay when a child fails to learn as expected—"What am I doing wrong?" Such feelings do not lead to appropriate referrals.

Another problem is that the paraprofessional may observe a child with a possible handicap but make a culturally appropriate rather than an educationally appropriate response. In some cultures, a child's problems are viewed as resulting from the actions of a distant past relative. To identify the child will bring shame upon the parents. Therefore, the paraprofessional never mentions such a problem.

In other cultures, handicaps are viewed as the result of punishment "from God" for unacceptable behaviors of the parents. The disapproved parental behaviors may range from infidelity to going outside when there was an eclipse (Meyerson, 1983). Again, however, the culturally appropriate response is for the paraprofessional to say nothing about the problem.

Finally, some cultures make accommodations or even provide recognition for certain handicaps. A deaf, communicatively disordered, mentally retarded, or mentally disturbed child can be maintained within many traditional societies in ways that either support the society or are minimally disruptive.

The school has an important responsibility in providing paraprofessionals with information to improve their understanding of the special programs available and of the school's orientation toward handicaps. Paraprofessionals need to be aware that no blame will be directed toward them for failing to educate the child and that the school will not blame the parents for the child's condition. By providing paraprofessionals with information about the nature of communicative disorders and the special services available to children who demonstrate these problems, the likelihood is increased that appropriate referrals will be made.

Paraprofessionals as Interpreters and Interviewers

When the parents of a child who has been referred for testing do not speak English, bilingual paraprofessionals may be the only personnel available locally who speak the language. A major problem in using paraprofessionals as interpreters is that they often are not familiar with the assessment process and with the educational concepts that need to be explained. A paraprofessional with no training in the field of special education, for example, would find it difficult to explain concepts such as *pragmatic language disorder, mainstreaming,* and *learning disability* to a parent who speaks only Vietnamese. Thus, training programs are needed to provide paraprofessionals with an understanding of educational terminology and the assessment process so that assessment forms, testing procedures, assessment results, and other pertinent information can be explained to the child's parents in a meaningful way.

In addition to serving in roles as interpreters, bilingual paraprofessionals can assist speech–language pathologists by conducting interviews with the child's parents. Juarez (1983) argued that trained interviewers rather than interpreters should be used when parents are interviewed to collect case history information. A trained interviewer was described by Juarez as "a person who has had formal training either through workshops or classes on how to conduct information-gathering interviews" (p. 58).

If paraprofessionals are to be used effectively in interviewing parents, they must be provided with the knowledge necessary to collect the information desired by the speech–language pathologist and other members of the assessment team. The specific questions that will be asked during the interviews should be explained to the paraprofessionals. They must understand the purpose of each question and must know how to record the interviewee's responses.

When trained paraprofessionals are used to interview parents, the speech–language pathologist should be available to answer any questions that may come up as the interview is being conducted. It is the speech–language pathologist's responsibility to make sure that the paraprofessional understands the information that needs to be conveyed to the child's parents and the information that needs to be obtained from them. This information always should be discussed in detail with the paraprofessional prior to any direct contact with the parents. Interviews conducted by the paraprofessional should be audiotaped, if at all possible, so that the content of the interview can be reviewed with the entire assessment team.

NEED FOR SALARIED BILINGUAL PARAPROFESSIONALS

Bilingual paraprofessionals hired for roles in bilingual education classrooms and in programs designed to teach English as a second language have provided valuable services for children from bilingual, bicultural backgrounds. The employment of salaried bilingual paraprofessionals specifically for roles in special education, however, has been limited.

Tolliver-Weddington and Meyerson (1983) stressed the need for salaried bilingual paraprofessionals in the field of speech–language pathology and argued that "often the seriousness of the role and continuity of the program is boosted by providing salaries rather than relying on volunteers' time" (p. 383). Paraprofessionals hired to serve under the direction of the speech–language pathologist can be provided with comprehensive, ongoing programs of in-service training that make it possible for them to serve in a variety of roles in both assessment and remediation. The increased use of salaried bilingual paraprofessionals in the field of speech–language pathology should facilitate the identification and appropriate educational placement of many bilingual, handicapped children in our schools.

CONCLUSION

The use of paraprofessionals in the assessment of bilingual children is a controversial issue. Educators, however, have both a legal and an ethical responsibility to provide all children with an equal opportunity for an appropriate education. School districts with populations of children who speak Samoan, Tagalog, Arabic, and other minority languages often do not have access to bilingual speech–language pathologists with the language fluency necessary to test these children. Should a school district with 250 Vietnamese-speaking students totally neglect the communicatively handicapped children in this population because there are no Vietnamese-speaking speech–language pathologists available to conduct the testing? When the services of a bilingual speech–language pathologist cannot be obtained, other alternatives must be considered or the needs of handicapped bilingual children will not be met.

Speech–language pathologists and other special educators must become involved in the development of strategies for training bilingual paraprofessionals to assist in the assessment of bilingual children. Paraprofessionals cannot replace speech–language pathologists, but the use of their services increases the likelihood that bilingual children with communicative disorders are identified and provided with appropriate remedial programs.

Chapter 4

Assessing Cultural and Environmental Influences

The world that the bilingual, bicultural child has experienced is often quite different from that experienced by members of the dominant culture. The conditions under which language is learned are largely culturally determined. Moreover, the form that social relations take varies from culture to culture, and differences are observed in the way language is used for communicative purposes. Cultural groups also differ in their values, mores, and in their interpretation of experiences. The cultural and environmental factors that may be having an impact on the child's communicative capabilities are important to consider in assessment.

LEARNING ABOUT OTHER CULTURES

Information needs to be obtained about the values, beliefs, experiences, and living conditions of the various cultural groups represented in the school setting if assessment data are to be collected and interpreted in a nonbiased manner. Speech–language pathologists, community aides, school psychologists, and other school personnel may participate in the collection of this information by "becoming anthropologists" and exploring the various cultures in the community. By interviewing community members from different cultural backgrounds, information can be gathered that should be helpful to school personnel in assessing the cultural and environmental factors that may be influencing children's performance in the school setting. It is also important to observe the behavior of individuals from different cultures both in the school and in various settings within the community.

Interviewing Bilingual, Bicultural Individuals

When interviewing individuals from a particular cultural background, it must be remembered that individual members of that group have had different experiences and, therefore, may not share identical cultural perspectives. For example, Vietnamese teenagers who were born in the United States and interact primarily with Anglo children may view their culture quite differently from Vietnamese individuals who are recent immigrants to this country. Similarly, discussions with Hispanic bilingual education teachers educated in the United States may reveal cultural perspectives different from those of Hispanic individuals who have never been provided with an opportunity for an education. Therefore, it is recommended that several individuals from each cultural group be interviewed so that differences in experiences within that culture can be examined.

The most readily available individuals to interview are those within the school setting. One can start by interviewing bilingual, bicultural teachers from the local community if any are available. Classroom instructional aides and other paraprofessionals working in the school setting are more likely than teachers to be from the local community. These individuals may have children in the school setting and often can provide useful insights about their culture. Students in junior and senior high school often have experienced a wide expanse of their culture and can provide valuable information to school personnel if selected carefully.

Community members who come into the school to serve on various school committees also can be interviewed. Each school that receives federal Title VII (bilingual) funds must have a bilingual advisory council that includes parents and community members. By interviewing members of school committees and observing these individuals as they interact with one another, much can be learned about the culture and the environment of the bilingual student population.

Outside of the school setting are additional sources of information. Soon after any ethnic group settles in a neighborhood, members of that group are likely to open churches and stores (Kincheloe, 1970). Church officials and grocery store merchants interact with parents and children on a regular basis and may provide information about the culture different from that acquired during interviews with individuals who have participated directly in school activities. Centers that offer special services for minority groups, newsstands, and hospitals are among the other potential locations where information about the various cultural groups in the community can be acquired.

Interviews should not be limited to bilingual, bicultural community members who are fluent speakers of English because these individuals are often the ones who have been influenced most by the Anglo culture. The most valuable information often is obtained from those who cannot communicate effectively in English. Therefore, it may be necessary to use interpreters when conducting interviews.

Questions to Ask about the Culture

Most limited English proficient children in the United States were born in this country (National Association of Bilingual Educators News, June, 1983). The cultural and environmental factors influencing the school performance of this group of children are often quite different from the factors influencing the performance of children who came to the United States to escape a crisis situation in their homeland. The specific questions that should be asked, therefore, vary depending on the background of the individual being interviewed. The following questions are among those that might be included when interviewing individuals to find out about their background and culture:

Why have members of the cultural group left their homeland? When the bilingual student population in the school setting includes children who immigrated to the United States from other countries, it is important to examine factors in the group's past that may have educational significance. Wars, oppressive regimes, and economic upheavals are among the reasons why many families have left their homeland. Families that have experienced poverty and starvation may have come to the United States in search of employment and better living conditions.

People travel long distances to escape war and persecution. Some families immigrate to the United States with few of their possessions. Moreover, it is not uncommon for some members of the family to be left behind.

Children in the school setting may have experienced trauma before or during the move to the United States. School personnel must be prepared to provide appropriate services for these children. Finding out about the history of the various cultural groups in the school setting is essential if school personnel are to understand their problems and their needs.

Why have members of the cultural group settled in the local community? The specific reasons why individuals from a particular cultural background have selected the local community as a place of residence should be examined. Some individuals may live in the local community because of community organizations that support their culture and religious beliefs. The availability of jobs may be another reason why the local community has been selected as a place of residence. Some families may have come to the local community because the housing available meets their needs.

Immigrants are likely to select a place of residence in the United States where some form of support is available to them. Eames and Goode (1977) reported that individuals tend to settle in areas where they have personal contacts with others. It is common for individuals to move to areas where they have both relatives and acquaintances (e.g., workmates, former schoolmates) with whom they continue to associate following the move (Denich, 1970). The assistance provided to immigrants when they first arrive in the community often comes from relatives and friends (Graves & Graves, 1974). Finding out about the patterns of support that are available to particular cultural groups within the community will provide insights about their way of life and about the specific problems that are being experienced.

To what extent is poverty experienced by members of the cultural group? Many immigrants and minority groups in the United States are living in extreme poverty. Migrant farm workers are at the bottom of the scale in terms of income, but even minority city workers often earn less than the minimum wage (Blackburn, 1983).

Stress, mental illness, and various physical problems can occur under extreme conditions of poverty (Wallis, 1983). When there are close-knit social relationships, the stress factors are reduced (Kleiner & Parker, 1975). Warmth, affection, and aid for major crises (e.g., long-term illness) typically come from kin and long-term friends (Roberts, 1974).

Two neighborhoods that are experiencing similar levels of poverty may provide quite different experiences and levels of support for the individuals within them (Trotter, 1974). The level of poverty experienced in the local community and the types of support available to individuals in times of extreme need should be examined.

What is the typical family size? The child-to-adult ratio may be quite high. Recent immigrants from war-torn countries (e.g., the "boat people") often have the children of deceased relatives living with them. In other groups, the number of people living in the home may continue to increase as additional relatives immigrate to the United States. Grandparents, cousins, and other relatives may all live in the same household. The number of people living in the home affects the type of interactions and learning opportunities that children experience.

What roles are assigned to individual family members? All of the *control* in some cultures is assigned to the elder members of the family. No decisions are made until these individuals, or sometimes the entire family, have been consulted. Young parents, in some cases, make *no* decisions themselves. Knowing the various roles of family members can help to explain why children behave the way they do in particular environments.

What customs, values and beliefs in the culture have relevance in understanding children's behavior? The rules governing how individuals are expected to act when interacting with others vary from culture to culture. Each culture has customs, values, and beliefs that influence the manner in which language is used for communicative purposes. Requesting that someone repeat an answer is acceptable within the Anglo culture but may be viewed as an insult in another culture. In some groups, individuals prefer not to answer a question on the same day that the question is asked (Hymes, 1971).

Cultural differences are reflected in both verbal and nonverbal patterns of communication. Vietnamese children, for example, show respect by avoiding eye contact when interacting with adults. These children may also smile when scolded by an individual senior in age or status (e.g., teachers) to indicate that they still have respect for that person (California State Department of Education, 1982). Vietnamese children tend to be reluctant to ask questions in class because such behavior is viewed as aggressive and disrespectful within their culture. They also may not volunteer answers during class because their culture expects them to be modest, polite, humble, and quiet (Wei, 1983).

Cultural differences observed among Native American children can be confused quite easily with communicative disorders. Children from various Native American groups, for example, may not answer questions posed by an adult who knows the answer to these questions. Thus, a Native American child may say nothing when asked to name pictures in a testing situation (G. Harris, 1983). Native American families tend to teach their children primarily through the visual modality. Visual awareness and highly developed observation skills are considered to be important by Native Americans. Native American children's strengths often lie in the visual rather than the verbal modality and these children may demonstrate restricted use of the spoken language in the classroom setting (Anderson & Anderson, 1983).

Bauman (1971) emphasized that "people of different societies think differently about language, value it differently, evaluate it differently, acquire it through different social mechanisms, use it in different situations, and turn it to different ends" (p. 335). Members of the assessment team must become sensitive to these cultural differences if they are to conduct assessments in a nondiscriminatory manner. Interviews with community members should be helpful to assessment personnel in identifying cultural differences that have relevance in the identification of children with communicative disorders.

What are the social functions and leisure activities in which members of the cultural group participate? Churches and other institutions may provide opportunities for individuals to socialize with other individuals from the same cultural background. There may be parties, marches, national sports (e.g., soccer), and other activities that provide opportunities for social interaction.

The extent to which members of the cultural group watch television, read books, and engage in various hobbies should also be examined. Their life style may differ in important respects from that of individuals from the Anglo culture.

How do members of the cultural group view the role of education? Many of the world's schools provide instruction using an authoritarian approach in which children are expected to follow rigid rules. Individuals from Vietnam who experienced the structured, lecture method of instruction used in that country may consider the open type of classroom in many American schools to be disorganized (Wei, 1983).

Some of the individuals interviewed may have never received an education and may have little awareness of what goes on in the school setting. Others may have expectations that are not being met within the educational program. It is important to find out about the value placed upon education within the culture and to identify specific concerns. This information is needed so that the school's program and special services can be explained to parents and so that culturally relevant programs can be developed.

How do members of the cultural group view handicapped individuals? Anglo parents often have hidden handicapped children out of sight. They may feel shame, embarrassment, and view the handicap as "their fault"—either something they have done or the result of "bad genes" within the family. Parents often find it difficult to accept the fact that they have a handicapped child.

The Anglo culture had, for many years, hidden handicapped children away in special classrooms, special schools, or in institutions. While the concept of *mainstreaming* has received much attention in the literature (Reynolds, 1962; Reynolds & Birch, 1982), it was not until the passage of PL 94-142 (1975) that programs to mainstream handicapped children were required. It literally took an Act of Congress to initiate changes in how these children were treated. The word *handicap* continues to carry a stigma within our society, although efforts are being made in the schools to change attitudes toward handicapped individuals.

Attitudes toward the handicapped vary from culture to culture. Some cultures may view a child's handicap as the result of a curse while others may attribute the handicap to fate. A parent may feel that the needs of the handicapped child can be met adequately within the culture and that special remedial services are not needed. In most Native American tribes, for example, mentally retarded children are "reluctantly, if at all, placed in training settings" (Anderson & Anderson, 1983, p. 170).

The social acceptability of behavior is an important factor in determining whether or not an individual has a handicap. The concept of normality is, in large part, culturally determined. Therefore, it is essential for assessment personnel to find out about the culture's perceptions of handicapped individuals and their attitudes about providing remediation for these handicaps.

CONSIDERATION OF INDIVIDUAL DIFFERENCES

Once assessment personnel have obtained information about the various cultural groups in the school setting, it should be easier to approach and work with individuals from bilingual, bicultural backgrounds. It should be stressed, however, that every child and family is unique. Not all members of a particular cultural group share the same experiences or follow the same customs. Individual members of the culture may differ in their religious beliefs and in the extent that they have been influenced by the Anglo culture. By interviewing community members, one is provided with some broad *stereotypes* about the community. It must not be assumed, however, that all members of a particular cultural group are the same. Each individual interacts in unique ways with the culture and with the environment—these differences must be considered in assessment. One can begin by collecting a detailed case history.

The Case History

The case history is one of the most important sources of data in the communication assessment of children from bilingual backgrounds. Behaviors identified as "abnormal" in the school setting often can be explained by the child's parents and may, in fact, be common among children within this particular culture.

The first step in obtaining case history information is to establish rapport with the parents. Questions asked by school personnel can be threatening and may infer that the school objects to the family's child-rearing practices. The parents should not feel that their privacy is being invaded. They must be informed of the reasons for the proposed assessment and must understand that the school is interested in helping their child.

Parents who have limited fluency in English should be interviewed in their native language. The services of bilingual paraprofessionals are often needed to assist monolingual school personnel in conducting the interviews. When paraprofessionals are used, the questions should be prepared in advance and discussed with them. Sample questions are presented in Appendix A.

Cultural Influences

The child's oral communication is influenced by the form that social relations take within the culture in which language was learned. Cultural groups differ from one another in the extent to which particular language functions are emphasized and in terms of how children are expected to behave during communicative interactions. In collecting the case history data, one needs to determine whether behaviors viewed as abnormal within the school setting are viewed in the same way within the child's culture. Information about the family's cultural customs, beliefs, child-rearing practices, and behavioral expectations for children can help clarify observations made within the school setting. Behaviors that are initially viewed as evidence of a communicative disorder by school personnel may, in many cases, be the result of differences in cultural expectations. A child should not be considered to have a communicative disorder if the behaviors observed are socially acceptable and occur frequently among children within the culture.

Environment and Language Exposure Patterns

The case history should include information about where, and under what circumstances, the child lived before arriving in the local community. The child may have experienced nutritional deficits, periods when meaningful communicative interactions were limited, and possible health hazards. A child's oral communication can be affected under conditions of stress. Emotional problems may result when a child leaves the homeland and must adjust to a new school and a new language. Among the factors that need to be explored are crises experienced by the family, reasons for leaving the homeland, the child's previous school history, and medical and developmental problems.

The family structure and the current conditions under which the family is living should also be examined. In cases of extreme poverty, it is not uncommon to find several families living under a single roof. Both parents may work long hours and have few opportunities to interact with their children. Often coupled with poverty is the occurrence of single-parent families. The child may have little or no contact with the parent who is not living in the home.

It is also important to identify language usage patterns in the home and local neighborhood. To what extent do the child's parents use the first and the second languages in the home? To what extent does the child use each language when interacting with parents, siblings, and neighborhood peers? One must also consider the amount of contact that the child has with various others in the home environment. Some children may spend most of the day with a babysitter or a relative who speaks a language different from that most often used by the parents. Presented below is a case study which illustrates the importance of examining language usage patterns in the home.

> Josefina, a 5-year-old Mexican-American child, was found to be both "limited English proficient" and "limited Spanish proficient" when administered a language dominance measure in her kindergarten classroom. The classroom teacher assumed that Spanish was the most appropriate language for this child's instructional program because the parents spoke only Spanish in the home. Josefina had no brothers or sisters.
>
> Because of her limited language proficiency and poor academic achievement in the classroom, Josefina was referred for an evaluation. The speech–language pathologist interviewed the parents and discovered that they worked long hours and that the child spent most of her time with an English-speaking babysitter. The parents also reported that the child seemed to prefer English when interacting with her bilingual peers.
>
> A comprehensive speech and language assessment revealed that Josefina's communication in both languages was characterized by limited vocabulary, word retrieval problems, poor sentence structure, auditory comprehension deficits, and multiple articulation errors. The test results also indicated that the child was English-dominant in all aspects of communication.

It would have been difficult to explain Josefina's dominance in the English language without information about the child's interactions with others in the home environment. Therefore, one must find out with whom the child interacts in various settings and the extent to which each language is used during those interactions.

A language usage form for estimating environmental exposure to both languages in various speaking contexts is illustrated on the following page. In this example, (S) (for subject) is placed along the continuum to indicate the extent to which the child uses the first language (L1) and the second language (L2) during interactions with each of the other individuals listed. An "X" is placed along the continuum to indicate the extent to which others speak each language to the child. The data in the matrix indicate that the child spoke the second language in most contexts (see Watson, Omark,

Name	Relationship	L1	Language Used L1 & L2 Equally	L2
Within home				
Pepe	Brother (older)			X (S)
Jorge	Father	X		(S)
Maria	Mother		X	(S)
Cecilia	Sister (older)			X(S)
Carlos	Uncle	X		(S)
Marta	Aunt		X	(S)
Tina	Niece (baby)	X	(S)	
Outside home				
Juan	Friend			X(S)
Jim	Friend			(S) X
Eddie	Friend			X (S)
Pete	Friend		X	(S)

Grouell, & Heller, 1981, for additional matrices that can be used to record observations).

The type of language model parents provide for the child and their attitudes toward use of the first and second languages should also be considered. Some parents encourage their children to use English in the home, whereas others prefer that only the native language be used. The child's development of language is influenced by the model provided by the parents, as shown in the following example.

> Pulu, a 5-year-old child, was referred for testing by his kindergarten teacher because of poor language structure and difficulty articulating English speech sounds. The child's parents were born in Samoa but have lived in the United States for 8 years. Pulu was born in Southern California and has never been outside of the United States.
>
> The speech–language pathologist spoke to Pulu's parents when they came for a conference with the classroom teacher. During the interview, it was learned that only English was used in the home with Pulu. The parents, however, often used Samoan when speaking to each other. Pulu's knowledge of Samoan was limited to a few words. The parents reported that Pulu's interactions in the home environment were primarily with family members and that the child did not play with other children in the neighborhood.
>
> Both parents had accents and demonstrated poor sentence structure when speaking English. It was observed that Pulu's speech and language patterns were similar to those used by his parents.

Because Pulu learned English from individuals who had limited proficiency in the language, one cannot expect him to be a fluent English speaker. Children learn the language as it is used in their environment, and their performance must be evaluated in relationship to that environment. Hence, it is necessary to examine the child's language environment before deciding that a communicative disorder is present.

CONCLUSION

People everywhere want their children to succeed but the paths to success can be very different (Perrone & Aleman, 1983). The collection of information about the bilingual child's culture can facilitate the development of appropriate strategies for both assessment and instructional programming. In particular, one should investigate how the various cultural groups in the local community perceive and care for their handicapped individuals. Some parents view handicaps as something that cannot be remediated and, therefore, may not understand why school personnel are interested in testing their child. Others may feel that the family rather than the school should be responsible for meeting the child's special needs. The success of the assessment team in developing an appropriate educational program for the child requires an understanding of cultural differences.

In addition to learning about the various cultural groups represented in the local community, one must also become aware of how individual families vary in their interactions with their culture. Some individuals manage to maintain their cultural heritage and their first language whereas others experience loss of both their cultural customs and their first language. Differences in experiences must be considered in assessment. By becoming anthropologists and gathering information about the various cultural groups represented in the local community, speech–language pathologists and other members of the assessment team are better equipped to meet the needs of children from bilingual, bicultural backgrounds.

Chapter 5

Published Tests and Their Limitations

Public Law 94-142 (1975) mandates that the assessment procedures used in the identification of handicapped children be culturally and linguistically appropriate. Therefore, when limited English proficient children are referred for speech–language assessments, it is necessary that testing be conducted in the dominant language. This chapter provides information about published tests for bilingual children and presents guidelines for the selection and use of these instruments.

PUBLISHED TESTS AND THE ASSESSMENT OF COMMUNICATIVE COMPETENCE

Most of the tests currently in use in the field of speech–language pathology are based on a structuralistic model of language. In such a model, language is viewed as a series of discrete points which, when added together, make the whole. Language proficiency tests reflecting this model are designed to examine the extent to which the child has mastered specific linguistic forms (grammatical forms, units of vocabulary, etc.). These tests are referred to as *discrete point tests* (Erickson, 1981).

The structuralistic view of language has been challenged in recent psycholinguistic and sociolinguistic research. Chomsky's (1965) theory on transformational generative grammar has stimulated an interest in studying children's development of a system of rules for the generation of utterances. Moreover, a theoretical shift has taken place in the field of speech–language pathology over the past decade as a result of research on the pragmatic aspects of communication. Bates (1976) defined pragmatics as "rules governing the use of language in context" (p. 420). When assessment is conducted within a pragmatic framework, communication is examined as it serves various functions in meaningful speaking contexts. This approach focuses on how communicative behavior varies as a function of the interactors, topic, and setting in which the interaction takes place.

A major limitation of discrete point tests in their failure to examine the child's competence in using language functionally for specific purposes. An interpersonal perspective is necessary when evaluating an individual's communicative competence.

> Competence lies in the relational system and as such must be evaluated from an interpersonal perspective. Cooperative discourse itself is a complex commitment to social interaction. This will mean that clinical assessment procedures which treat language competencies as fixed, with little or no reference to the relational system, need to be questioned. (Prutting, 1982, p. 129)

Discrete point tests often require the child to perform tasks that require psychological operations different from those required in natural speaking contexts. Oller (1983; see also Oller, 1979) argued that two pragmatic naturalness criteria must be considered in the evaluation of test items. First, test items must not violate the normal temporal development of discourse. Second, test items must have a meaningful connection to ordinary experience. The problems that can result when these pragmatic naturalness constraints are violated were described by Oller (1983) as follows:

> The pragmatic naturalness constraints reflect respectively the temporal development and the usual meaningfulness of discourse. Tests that analyze language in ways that destroy these ordinary properties of discourse probably are not very good language tests. They may invoke *aspects* of language skills but will probably do so only superficially. More important, such tests generally will lack construct validity. (p. 81)

Although the use of discrete point tests has been challenged, these measures continue to be used in most bilingual settings (Day, McCollum, Cieslak, & Erickson, 1981). Test instruments that focus solely on the structural aspects of language provide a limited picture of the child's performance capabilities. Instruments designed to assess children's ability to use language functionally are urgently needed.

Discrete point tests, in spite of their limitations, can provide information that may be helpful in identifying specific areas of deficit demonstrated by children with communicative disorders. These tests, however, should always be used in conjunction with measures of the child's functional use of language during natural communication activities (see chap. 6). Measurement of the child's communicative competence as language is used for various purposes in natural speaking contexts should be the primary area of emphasis in assessment.

ARTICULATION TESTS

Articulation tests are used to assess the child's production of the speech sounds of the language. Sounds may be assessed in isolation, nonsense syllables, words, sentences, reading, or conversation. Articulation tests that assess production of isolated words generally elicit responses using tasks in which the child is asked to repeat words, finish incomplete sentences, or name pictures.

English Articulation Tests

Most published English articulation tests use picture-naming tasks to elicit production of the phonemes of the language in the initial, medial, and final position of words. The Fisher–Logemann Test of Articulation Competence (Fisher & Logemann, 1971), Templin–Darley Test of Articulation (Templin & Darley, 1960), and the Weiss Comprehensive Articulation Test (Weiss, 1978) are among the tests available that use this approach. The information obtained from these measures is used to identify the specific phonemes that the child is unable to produce correctly. These instruments are based on the phonological system of Standard American English and were standardized on native English speakers. Use of these tests can result in misdiagnosis if Anglo norms are used in interpreting assessment data obtained on children from bilingual, bicultural backgrounds. These tests, however, can be useful in assessing bilingual children's progress in acquiring the phonology of the second language.

Articulation Tests in Languages Other than English

Few published articulation tests are available in languages other than English. Recently, several articulation tests have become available in Spanish. These include the Austin Spanish Articulation Test (Carrow, 1974), the Southwestern Spanish Articulation Test (Toronto, 1972), and the Medida Espanola de Articulación (La "Meda") (Mason, Smith, & Henshaw, 1976). A survey conducted by Mattes (1982c) revealed that the Austin Spanish Articulation Test was the instrument most frequently used by speech–language pathologists in Los Angeles County to assess the articulation of Spanish speakers. The only Spanish articulation test that provides normative data is the Medida Española de Articulación.

All three of the Spanish articulation measures mentioned above are designed for use in assessing children's production of individual speech sounds at the word level. These tests assess phoneme production without regard to context and do not provide sufficient information to determine the influence of factors such as stress patterns or syllable types. Moreover, none of these tests provides procedures for using the assessment data to identify the phonological processes that characterize the child's speech.

The dialect spoken by the child is an important consideration in determining the appropriateness of an articulation test for local use. The verbal stimuli used on the test must be familiar to the child. Moreover, the extent to which the test content is representative of the phonological structure of the child's dialect needs to be examined (Iglesias, 1983). If an articulation test is used that was not developed locally, assessment personnel must be able to identify those items that are not appropriate for local use so that children are not penalized for dialect differences.

Articulation Testing and Phonological Processes

Formal articulation tests serve a valuable function in assessment because they make it possible to sample specific aspects of the child's phonological behavior in a systematic manner. These measures, however, generally do not provide sufficient information to assess the systematicity of the child's misarticulations.

The individual articulation errors produced by children often reflect general phonological processes such as syllable deletion, consonant cluster reduction, final consonant deletion, and assimilation (Hodson & Paden, 1983; Ingram, 1976). Phonemes need to be examined in a variety of contexts so that patterns of error that occur across phonemes can be identified. The results of formal articulation tests should always be supplemented by data obtained from connected speech samples and from informal measures of phonological production. Procedures for the analysis of phonological processes have been described in the literature (Hodson & Paden, 1983; Weiner, 1979).

TESTS OF LANGUAGE DOMINANCE

Tests of language dominance are designed for use in measuring an individual's relative linguistic proficiency in two languages. Whether or not a bilingual child is placed in a bilingual program of instruction is often determined from the results of these measures. These results are used by assessment personnel in special education to identify those students who need to be tested in a language other than English. Special education personnel need information on language dominance "primarily to avoid the misdiagnosis (and subsequent misplacement) of non-native English-speaking students and to identify language deficiencies which need attention" (DeBlassie, 1980, p. 46).

A variety of approaches have been used in the assessment of language dominance. One commonly used approach is to assess the child's relative proficiency in the vocabulary of the two languages. The James Language Dominance Test (James, 1974), for example, focuses on assessing the child's comprehension and production of vocabulary in English and Spanish. The receptive portion of this test consists primarily of items that require the child to point to a picture named by the examiner; most of the items on the expressive portion require the child to name pictures. Only 2 of the 40 items on this test requires more than a one-word response.

In contrast to the James Language Dominance Test, the Bilingual Syntax Measure (Burt, Dulay, & Hernandez-Chavez, 1976) focuses entirely on assessing the child's syntactic abilities. Performance is assessed in English and Spanish based on the child's responses to questions asked about cartoon-like pictures. The test is designed to elicit natural speech which is then measured for syntactic proficiency. The authors of the test argue that syntax is the most suitable measure of proficiency because it shows less variation across dialects and idiolects than pronunciation, vocabulary, or measures of functional language use.

> Of the various characteristics of a particular language, syntax shows the least variation among speakers of the language. Most research in child language acquisition focuses on syntax and, as a result, descriptions of syntactic developmental sequences provide invaluable input for the assessment of language development. (Burt et al., 1976, p. 10)

When language dominance tests are used, assessment personnel must be aware that dominance can vary depending on the specific aspect of language that is being assessed (Burt & Dulay, 1978). A child who is dominant in the syntax of the first language, for example, may be dominant in the vocabulary of the second language. Therefore, the testing of language dominance should consider how performance varies depending on what is being assessed.

The Language Assessment Scales (DeAvila & Duncan, 1977) have become popular as a language dominance measure in bilingual education programs because they assess a variety of aspects of the child's language behavior. The test includes subtests that measure sound discrimination, phoneme production, vocabulary, sentence comprehension, and oral production (storytelling). The level of proficiency in each language is determined from the child's total score. A major weakness of this test is that the sample of behavior obtained from each subtest is quite limited. Therefore, use of this measure to determine how the child's dominance varies in different aspects of the language is not recommended.

The validity of published language dominance tests for use in assessing bilingual children's ability to function effectively in school has been questioned. Cummins (1981) has argued that tests must have predictive validity for academic achievement if they are to be of value in the educational placement of bilingual children. Some measures, according to Cummins, are designed specifically *not* to relate to achievement in an academic setting (e.g., the Bilingual Syntax Measure). Many of the language dominance tests were published without data on their reliability and validity (Silverman, Noa & Russell, 1976; Watson, Omark, Grouell, & Heller, 1981). Without such information, one has no way of knowing whether these tests are measuring what they were designed to measure.

If a language dominance test is valid, one would expect performance on the measure to correlate highly with performance during conversational speech. The performance of 32 Mexican-American children on three language dominance tests and tape-recorded samples of conversational speech in English and Spanish was examined in a study conducted by Gerken (1978). The tests used were the James Language Dominance Test, Comprehension of Oral Language Test, and the Dos Amigos Verbal Language Scales. Gerken found that there were significant correlations between the language dominance tests. Evaluators' ratings of the conversational samples, however, did not correlate highly with the results of these tests. Thus, language dominance as measured by structured tasks may not be a valid predictor of language dominance as measured during conversational speech.

Discrete-Point Dominance versus Functional Competence

In the assessment of language dominance, it is not as important to examine how much of each language the child knows as it is to evaluate the child's ability to operate *effectively* in each language in meaningful speaking contexts. The discrete-point language dominance tests, the measures most often used in our schools, focus solely on the structural aspects of language and, therefore, do not achieve this purpose. Whenever language dominance tests are administered, the results should be used in conjunction with data obtained from natural communication samples and other measures (see Erickson and Omark, 1981).

Questionnaires completed by relevant others in the child's environment are frequently used to identify the language in which the child communicates most effectively. The Home Bilingual Usage Estimate (Skoczylas, 1971), for example, is completed by the child's parents and examines the extent to which English and Spanish are used by the child and other individuals in the home environment. The instrument yields a single score that is used to classify children into one of the following categories: (1) English monolingual, (2) English dominant, (3) apparent bilingual, (4) Spanish dominant, (5) Spanish monolingual.

Estimates of the extent to which the child uses each language in various settings are not necessarily valid predictors of the child's relative proficiency in using the two languages (Teitelbaum, 1977). Walters (1979) argued that these measures "often confuse language dominance with language preference" (p. 4). Examining the extent to which each language is used tells one nothing about the child's effectiveness as a communicator. The child's communicative effectiveness in each language should be measured using information obtained from natural communication samples and interviews with the child's parents and others.

NORM-REFERENCED TESTS OF LANGUAGE PROFICIENCY

Many of the published language tests used in the field of speech–language pathology provide data that make it possible to compare an individual child's performance with that of other children the same age. The results of these tests are often used as a basis for determining whether or not children qualify for enrollment in remedial speech–language programs.

Tests of English Language Proficiency

Most norm-referenced tests of English language proficiency were standardized on a sample that consisted primarily of Anglo children. A common approach in the development of test norms is to select individuals from various strata of the national population based on each strata's representation in that population. Tests developed using this approach are likely to have a normative sample consisting of about 85% Anglo children with the remaining children representing various minority groups. Therefore, the norms will reflect most accurately the performance of Anglo children and may not be valid when used with other groups (Omark, 1981a).

Mattes (1982c) found that the tests most often used by speech–language pathologists in Los Angeles County to assess the English language proficiency of Spanish-speaking children were the Del Rio Language Screening Test, Test for Auditory Comprehension of Language, Peabody Picture Vocabulary Test, Northwestern Syntax Screening Test, and the Illinois Test of Psycholinguistic Abilities. With the exception of the Del Rio Language Screening Test, all of these tests were standardized on samples that consisted primarily of Anglo children. Use of these norms to interpret the performance of minority children from bilingual backgrounds is not appropriate.

The following case illustrates the problems that can occur when norms from tests standardized on monolingual English-speaking children are used in evaluating the performance of children from bilingual backgrounds.

> Tone, a 7-year-old Samoan child, was referred for a speech–language assessment because of poor communication skills in English. Samoan was the language spoken most often in the home during the first 5 years of Tone's life. His parents began to speak only English in the home when Tone entered kindergarten because they wanted him to succeed in an English-speaking classroom. Although Tone was more proficient in Samoan than in English when he entered kindergarten, English is now his dominant language.
>
> The speech–language assessment was conducted in English, the child's dominant language, using the Peabody Picture Vocabulary Test and the Illinois Test of Psycholinguistic Abilities. Tone demonstrated more than a 2-year delay on both of these tests.
>
> The speech–language pathologist concluded that Tone had a language disorder based on the delay demonstrated on the norm-referenced tests. Enrollment in a remedial speech–language program was recommended.

The speech–language pathologist in the case described above failed to consider the child's language history in the interpretation of the test results. This child has had less experience in using the English language than has the typical monolingual English speaker. Moreover, a variety of cultural factors may have accounted for specific difficulties demonstrated by the child on the language measures.

Bilingual children who speak English as their dominant language need to be tested in English but are not necessarily handicapped when their performance falls significantly below the norm for monolingual English-speaking children. The extent to which the child has been exposed to the language and the influence of cultural and linguistic differences need to be considered (Briere, 1972; Cazden, 1973; Leeman, 1981).

Tests of Proficiency in Languages Other Than English

When bilingual children are referred for speech–language evaluations, assessment data are needed in both of the child's languages. A variety of language tests have been published for use in the assessment of Spanish-speaking children. There are few test instruments available, however, for speakers of minority languages other than Spanish.

Translations of English Tests

Translations of English language tests are often used in the assessment of children from bilingual backgrounds. The fact that a test has been shown to be valid in English does not necessarily mean that the test is valid when translated into other languages. The case that follows illustrates a situation commonly encountered when translations of English tests are used.

> Maria, a 6-year-old Spanish-speaking child with limited English proficiency, was referred for a language evaluation by her classroom teacher. A Spanish translation of the Peabody Picture Vocabulary Test was administered to assess her understanding of vocabulary. Using the norms provided in the manual for the English version of the test, Maria scored at the 10th percentile. The speech–language pathologist concluded that the child had a receptive language delay.

In the above example, English test norms were used to interpret data obtained when a Spanish translation of the Peabody Picture Vocabulary Test was used. The difficulty level of test items, however, is likely to change when an English test is translated into another language. Thus, a concept that is familiar to most English-speaking Anglo children at 5 years of age is not necessarily familiar to most 5-year-old children when translated into Spanish. Children from different cultures come to school with different experiences and their performance on tests reflects those experiences (DeBlassie & Franco, 1983). English test norms are valid *only* for the English version of the test and, therefore, should never be used when the test is translated into other languages.

A major problem in translating tests is that many English concepts do not have an exact equivalent in other languages. A concept that can be expressed in a single word in English may require two or more words when translated into another language. Efforts to produce literal translations of tests can result in test items that do not reflect the language as it is experienced by young children in their natural environment.

Translations of English tests often fail to tap critical linguistic features that need to be assessed in the child's language. The linguistic structures of languages differ and these differences need to be considered in assessment (Burt & Dulay, 1978). The Spanish language, for example, classifies all nouns as either masculine or feminine. In forming sentences, articles and adjectives must agree in gender with the noun. The masculine article form *el*, for example, and the masculine adjective form *viejo* are used in the phrase *el libro viejo* (the old book) so that they agree in gender with the masculine noun *libro*. Likewise, the feminine article form *la* and the feminine adjective form *vieja* are used in the phrase *la casa vieja* (the old house) so that they agree in gender with the feminine noun *casa*. This important structural aspect of the Spanish language does not exist in English and, therefore, is not tested when Spanish translations of English tests are used.

Tests must reflect the structure of the child's language if they are to provide valid assesment data. The Spanish version of the Test for Auditory Comprehension of Language (Carrow, 1973) illustrates many of the problems commonly experienced when Spanish translations of English tests are used. This test is a standardized measure of receptive language consisting of 101 parallel items in English and Spanish. The instrument is designed for children between 3 and 6 years of age.

The test manual provides limited information about the procedures used in developing the Spanish translation of the test. The Spanish version was field-tested on Spanish-speaking children, but normative data are available only for the English version of the test.

Rueda and Perozzi (1977) compared 20 children's performance on the Spanish translation of the Test for Auditory Comprehension of Language with their performance on the Screening Test of Spanish Grammar. The Screening Test of Spanish Grammar was developed specifically for use in assessing Spanish-speaking children. The researchers found that the correlation between 24 syntactical structures common to both tests was not significant. Syntactical structures were produced in error more often on the Test for Auditory Comprehension of Language than on the Screening Test of Spanish Grammar. Rueda and Perozzi suggested that the nonsignificant correlation between the two tests may have resulted because the Test for Auditory Comprehension of Language is a translation from English while the Screening Test of Spanish Grammar is derived directly from the Spanish language.

An analysis of test items on the Spanish version of the Test for Auditory Comprehension of Language revealed that problems with the translation may have affected the performance of the subjects tested. The translation for *farmer*, for example, was *ranchero* without the qualifying article *el*. Children may experience confusion on test items in which the necessary articles are omitted, because articles are important in conveying meaning in Spanish.

Questions regarding the diagnostic usefulness of the Spanish version of the Test for Auditory Comprehension of Language were also raised by Day et al. (1981). They reported that some of the test items represent only the Mexican form of Spanish. Therefore, users of the test must be able to identify items that may be linguistically inappropriate for the local student population.

Moreover, the relationship between the test items and developmental information on the Spanish language has not been investigated.

The Boehm Test of Basic Concepts (Boehm, 1971) is another popular norm-referenced test that has been translated into Spanish. The instrument assesses understanding of 50 concepts considered essential for achievement in the primary school years. This test was designed as a screening and teaching tool for children in kindergarten, first, and second grade.

The English version of the test has been criticized because of problems in selecting test content, inadequacies in the selection of the norming sample, and lack of sufficient information on the instrument's validity (Day et al., 1981). Because of these limitations, Day et al. argued that "one can only question the use of a Spanish translation" (p. 151).

The Spanish version of the test is a direct translation of the English version. Some of the concepts tested, however, do not have an exact equivalent in both languages. The concept *nearest*, for example, cannot be translated into Spanish in a single word. Therefore, the two words *mas cerca* are used to convey this concept on the Spanish version of the test. No information is reported about the difficulty level of individual items on the Spanish translation. Therefore, it cannot be assumed that the English and Spanish versions of this test are equivalent in difficulty.

Normative data are not available for the Spanish version of this test. Moreover, the reliability and validity of the Spanish translation have not been studied. Further research on this instrument is needed before it can be used with confidence in assessing children's comprehension of basic concepts.

The Test for Auditory Comprehension of Language and the Boehm Test of Basic Concepts exemplify some of the limitations inherent in the use of translations of English language tests. Translations are likely to be of minimal diagnostic value if they do not reflect children's cultural experiences or the important structural components of their language. Therefore, assessment personnel must be aware of the limitations of these measures so that test results are not misused.

Tests Normed on Bilingual Student Populations

A variety of norm-referenced Spanish language tests have become available, but little progress has been made in the development of tests for speakers of other minority languages. The norm-referenced Spanish language tests are all discrete-point measures designed to assess specific structural aspects of the language. Descriptions of some of the most widely used tests are presented in Appendix B.

It has been argued that nationally normed tests need to be developed for the various languages spoken by minority groups in this country. These norms would make it possible to compare a child's performance with that of a national sample of children who speak the same language. The development of nationally normed tests valid for all bilingual children is unrealistic, however, because of the heterogeneity of the various bilingual groups in this country.

> The most common suggestion for testing minorities centers around the creation of a comprehensive, nationally normed test for each minority. This is an interesting proposition but it is probably impossible to create such a normed test for many behaviors. To create an appropriate nationally normed test, one must have a homogeneous national group to standardize it. Minority groups vary tremendously from region to region and sometimes within the same community. (Toronto & Merrill, 1983, p. 105)

The development of nationally normed tests is difficult because of the many variations in dialect that can be found in different parts of the country. The Spanish dialect used by Mexican Americans, for example, is different from that used by Cuban Americans. Moreover, Mexican Americans in San Diego, California speak a dialect different from that used in Del Rio, Texas or Chicago, Illinois. It is unrealistic to assume that a single, nationally normed test is unbiased for all speakers of a particular language.

An alternative to the use of nationally normed tests is to use tests developed and normed in the local community. Locally normed tests make it possible to compare children with peers who have had similar experiences (Toronto & Merrill, 1983; Watson, Omark, Grouell, & Heller, 1981). The Screening Test of Spanish Grammar (Toronto, 1973), Del Rio Language Screening Test (Toronto, Leverman, Hanna, Rosenzweig, & Maldonado, 1975), and Pruebas de Expresión Oral y Percepción de la Lengua Española (Mares, 1980) are among the Spanish language tests that were normed on localized populations. In addition to providing local norms, these tests were written to reflect the local dialect.

A major problem with many of the norm-referenced tests available for Spanish-speaking children is that they provide limited information about the subject sample used in test standardization. The Prueba del Desarrollo Inicial del Lenguaje (Hresko, Reid, & Hammill, 1982), for example, presents separate norms for the United States, Mexico, and Puerto Rico but no information is provided about the criteria used in selecting children for the norming sample. Factors such as community of residence, place of birth, age of arrival in the United States, and language most often used in the home are not reported for Spanish-speaking children in the United States who participated in the norming of the test. Without such information it is impossible to judge the adequacy of the norming sample as a comparison group for individual children who are administered the test. Test norms should not be used if the test manual fails to provide a detailed description of the test standardization sample.

When language minority children are referred for testing and there are no appropriate norm-referenced tests available, assessment personnel must rely entirely on assessment data obtained from other sources. Criterion-referenced tests, conversational communication samples, and observational checklists are among the alternative approaches that can be used in the identification of bilingual children with communicative disorders (see chap. 6).

TESTS FOR APHASIA

The term *aphasia* is used to describe "an impairment of language functioning of persons who have incurred localized cerebral damage that results in a reduced likelihood that an individual involved in a communicative situation will understand or produce appropriate verbal formulations" (Eisenson, 1971, p. 1220). Common causes of aphasia include strokes, tumors, and traumatic injuries to the brain. Impairments resulting from aphasia are observed to affect listening, speaking, reading, and writing. Auditory comprehension deficits, word retrieval problems, inappropriate word substitutions, perseveration, and poor speech intelligibility are among the symptoms commonly observed when individuals acquire communicative disorders following brain injury. Aphasic individuals often experience difficulty recalling names for common nouns; related words may be substituted (e.g., *fork* substituted for *knife*). Moreover, the word-finding problems of aphasic individuals tend to vary under different stimulus conditions. Aphasia may be accompanied by other impairments such as *oral verbal apraxia*, an inability to make voluntary and purposeful movements of the articulatory mechanism.

A variety of approaches have been used in tests designed to assess the nature and severity of communicative disorders resulting from aphasia. The Language Modalities Test for Aphasia (Wepman & Jones, 1961) is based on the assumption that aphasic impairments are modality bound disturbances that are differentially classifiable. The results of this test are used to classify individuals as having pragmatic aphasia, semantic aphasia, syntactic aphasia, jargon aphasia, or global aphasia. The Minnesota Test for Differential Diagnosis of Aphasia (Schuell, 1965), on the other hand, is based on the assumption that aphasia manifests itself across all modalities. Schuell's major classifications of aphasic impairment are derived from the overall pattern of deficits observed. Assessment personnel should consider the theoretical framework underlying test development when selecting instruments for local use.

Tests used in the assessment of aphasia also differ in the methods used in scoring responses. Some tests focus only on the accuracy of the individual's responses while others consider qualitative variables. The Porch Index of Communicative Ability (Porch, 1967) uses a 16-point multidimensional scoring system in which individual responses are measured in terms of their accuracy, completeness, responsiveness, promptness, and efficiency.

An aphasia test for Spanish speakers that is available in an experimental edition is the Examines Para Diagnosticar Impedimentos de Afasia (Moncada & Marshall, 1982). This test, a Spanish adaptation of the Aphasia Language Performance Scales (Keenan & Brassell, 1975), assesses listening, speaking, reading, and writing. The test manual provides no information about the procedures used in developing the Spanish version of the instrument. Spanish adaptations of other tests have been developed but, to our knowledge, are not commercially available.

When bilingual individuals with aphasia are assessed, manifestations of the disorder should be identified in both the native language and in English. Cases have been reported in which the symptoms of aphasia observed in the first language were different from those observed in the second language (Albert & Obler, 1978). To assess the severity of aphasia, speech–language pathologists need to obtain information about the individual's previous ability to listen, speak, read, and write in each language. Family members and relevant others in the individual's environment should be interviewed to obtain this information.

The behavior of aphasic individuals on tests is likely to vary depending on the stimulus materials used and the manner in which the instrument is constructed. Moreover, the specific error types produced by aphasics on structured tasks may be very different from those produced during conversational speech (Mattes, 1976). The performance of bilingual individuals with aphasia should, therefore, be assessed in both languages under a variety of stimulus conditions.

In addition to assessing performance on formal listening, speaking, reading, and writing tasks, the effect of the impairment on the individual's functional use of each language should be examined. Family members, for example, may have noticed changes in the extent to which the individual makes use of each language in various speaking contexts since the onset of the disorder. Albert and Obler (1978) reported cases of bilingual aphasics who demonstrated "a mixing problem, combining elements of words or sentences from each language" (p. 151).

We have observed Spanish speakers with aphasia who produced utterances during conversation in which there were frequent alternations between English and Spanish. In contrast to the grammatical nature of the code switching behavior observed among normal bilingual speakers, however, the code switching observed among aphasic individuals often resulted in utterances that were ungrammatical. Moreover, these utterances often appeared to be devoid of meaning. We have observed other Spanish-speaking aphasics who switched to English when unable to retrieve an appropriate Spanish word. The assessment of communication in context is necessary to determine how the disorder manifests itself in each language and to identify the strategies used by the individual to convey specific communicative intents.

In the absence of an adequate battery of aphasia assessment instruments designed specifically for bilingual speakers, speech–language pathologists must rely on adapted versions of existing tests or on locally developed measures. Most of the published aphasia tests are designed for use in assessing individuals who had fully mastered basic speaking and literacy skills prior to brain injury and, therefore, are not appropriate for young children. Tests selected for use in the assessment of aphasia should be age-appropriate for the children being assessed. When translations of English aphasia tests are used, modifications should be made as necessary to reflect the cultural and linguistic experiences of the local population.

TESTS FOR THE HEARING IMPAIRED

When bilingual children with hearing impairments are assessed, the effect of the auditory impairment on oral communication must be examined. Speech audiometry measures are more important than pure tone thresholds in understanding the functional effects of the hearing impairment (Cooper, 1983). Measures of the hearing-impaired child's speech reception threshold and speech discrimination ability are essential components of the audiological evaluation.

Speech reception threshold tests used in the assessment of English-speaking children generally use spondaic words as test stimuli. Spondaic words are two syllables in length and have equal stress on each syllable (e.g., *baseball*). The words are presented to the individual through earphones. The level at which half of the words are repeated correctly is the speech reception threshold (Cooper, 1983; Davis, 1970).

The vocabulary words used in assessing the speech reception threshold must be familiar to the child being tested. Therefore, the use of English word lists in assessing the limited English proficient child is likely to produce invalid results. Limited English proficient children should be assessed in their native language so that their chances for success are maximized.

The use of spondaic words is inappropriate for languages that have stress patterns different from those used in English. Speech reception testing in Spanish, for example, can best be accomplished by the use of trochaic words in which the first syllable is stressed and the second syllable is unstressed. These words reflect the stress patterns most often used in the Spanish language (De Leon Northrup, 1983). A prerecorded speech reception threshold test for Spanish speakers that can be administered by individuals who do not speak Spanish is available (Martin & Hart, 1978).

Once the child's speech reception threshold has been determined, speech discrimination testing can begin. Tests of speech discrimination available for hearing-impaired English speakers generally use monosyllabic words as stimuli. These word lists are designed so that all of the phonemes of the language are represented. The individual's task is to repeat words presented at some level above (e.g., 40 dB) the speech reception threshold (Cooper, 1983; Davis, 1970).

The use of monosyllabic words is appropriate in the assessment of English speakers because of the large number of monosyllabic words in the language. Other languages, however, have few monosyllabic words and, therefore, must make use of words more than one syllable in length. Speech discrimination tests for Spanish speakers generally have used trocaic words (De Leon Northrup, 1983). Monosyllabic nonsense syllables have also been used in the speech discrimination testing of Spanish speakers (Ferrer, 1960).

Published word lists designed for use in assessing speech reception thresholds and speech discrimination are not available in many of the languages spoken by children in this country. Therefore, the local development of such measures often becomes necessary when limited English proficient children are assessed. Audiologists need to work closely with native speakers of the child's language so that linguistically appropriate word lists can be developed. Additional issues in the audiological screening and assessment of bilingual children are reviewed by Cooper (1983; see also Stewart, 1983).

USING TESTS TO IDENTIFY COMMUNICATIVE DISORDERS: A NONBIASED APPROACH

The previous sections of this chapter have provided an overview of the types of tests available for use in the speech and language assessment of bilingual, bicultural student populations. A major problem faced by assessment personnel is that of selecting test instruments that yield nonbiased data. Bias in assessment, however, is not limited to the test instruments used in data collection. Rather, the bias that occurs in assessment often reflects the way test data are interpreted and used (Bailey & Harbin, 1980; Duffey, Salvia, Tucker, & Ysseldyke, 1981). The remainder of this chapter offers practical strategies and guidelines for selecting, administering, and interpreting speech and language tests in a nondiscriminatory manner.

Selection of Appropriate Tests

A test evaluation form designed for use in reviewing the adequacy of published test instruments for local use is presented in Appendix C. This form is completed based on a careful reading of the examiner's manual, a review of the test format and the content of individual test items, and information obtained when the instrument is field-tested on children from the local population. In addition to providing a system for rating tests in eight specific areas, the evaluation form provides space for comments. Thus, specific problems in the test content, administration procedures, cultural appropriateness of test items, and so forth, can be recorded. The eight areas included on the test evaluation form are summarized below.

1. Purposes of the test. The test manual should be reviewed to determine the specific purposes for which the test is designed. Not all language tests are designed for use in the identification of children with communicative disorders. If the test manual specifies that the test is designed for use as a screening tool, then it should be used only for that purpose. Misdiagnosis is likely if tests are used for purposes other than those for which they were intended.

2. Construction of the test. The theoretical model underlying the development of the test and the procedures used in test construction (e.g., item selection) should be examined. As mentioned earlier, most tests are based on structural linguistic theory rather than current theories that focus on the functional aspects of communication (Erickson, 1981). The extent to which the test was field-tested prior to standardization is also an important diagnostic consideration.

3. Procedures. Procedures for test administration, scoring, and interpretation should be described in detail in the test manual. The extent to which these procedures are appropriate for local use needs to be considered. The length of the test, examiner qualifications necessary for test administration, and the complexity of the scoring system are among the factors that should be examined in selecting tests that are appropriate for the local population.

4. Linguistic appropriateness of the test. The use of speech and language tests designed specifically for speakers of a particular language does not guarantee that the linguistic content of these instruments is appropriate for all children who speak that language. Dialect differences must be considered in the selection of tests. Spanish words for *hot, jacket,* and *banana*, for example, are among those that vary in different dialects. Thus, one can be penalized for not having been exposed to the dialect used on the test (Burt & Dulay, 1978; Ortiz, 1980).

It is recommended that a minimum of two native adult speakers of the language who are fluent in the local dialect be involved in the review of test content. They should also participate in the review of data obtained when the instrument is field-tested locally. Test items that are responded to incorrectly by a large percentage of the children should be examined carefully in terms of their linguistic appropriateness.

5. Cultural appropriateness of test items. The ability to respond correctly to test items often requires an experiential projection into the situation in question. Some individuals, for example, might be likely to select *coat* as being associated with *snow* rather than selecting *toboggan* because of their experiential background with these concepts (Cervantes, 1974). Therefore, test instruments should be reviewed by native speakers of the language and field-tested to identify items that may be culturally inappropriate for the local population.

The testing materials (e.g., illustrations presented to the child) and test administration procedures also should be evaluated in terms of their cultural appropriateness. Illustrations used to elicit responses from the child may depict situations that have never been experienced by children from the local school population. Moreover, the test may require the performance of tasks that violate cultural norms concerning the way children are expected to behave when interacting with an adult. When children are asked to perform culturally inappropriate tasks, they may exhibit behavior that seems abnormal to individuals who are not familiar with their culture.

6. Adequacy of norms. The examiner's manual should provide a detailed description of the criteria used in selecting children for the standardization sample. This sample must be an appropriate comparison group for children in the local population if the normative data are to be useful in test interpretation. Factors such as ethnic background, socioeconomic level, place of birth, length of residency in the United States, language most often used in the home, and language classification (e.g., limited English proficient) need to be considered. If the test manual does not provide a detailed description of the specific procedures used in selecting children for the standardization sample, the validity of the norms for local use must be questioned.

7. Adequacy of test reliability data. Reliability refers to the extent to which a test *consistently* yields the same results. A test with high reliability results in scores that are about the same from one test administration to the next if a similar population is assessed. Tests with reliability coefficients below .80 should be considered inadequate (see Watson, Omark, Grouell, & Heller, 1981).

8. Adequacy of test validity data. A test with high reliability is not necessarily a valid instrument. Validity refers to the extent to which a test measures what it is designed to measure. A test that has been validated only as a language dominance measure is not necessarily valid for use in determining whether or not a child demonstrates a communicative disorder. Therefore, the validity data reported in the test manual should be examined to determine if the instrument has been validated for all of its intended uses.

Because of the limited availability of speech and language tests for bilingual populations, school districts may find that there are no tests that will meet the needs of students in the local community. Three procedures were suggested by Evard and Sabers (1979) which can be used in efforts to improve the validity of speech and language test data obtained from distinct ethnic–racial groups:

1. The development of a new test. Tests can be developed locally to ensure that test content is relevant to the linguistic and cultural background of the students being tested. Test construction, however, is time consuming and may not be cost effective if the assessment instrument is developed for a small student population.

2. The adaptation of an existing test. An existing test may be adapted so as to be appropriate for use in assessing individuals from a specific ethnic–racial group. When such changes are introduced, however, new norms must be developed.

3. The development of local test norms. Local test norms may be developed for existing tests by administering these tests to a representative sample of students from the local student population. The development of local test norms, however, does not guarantee that the test is *valid* for local use.

The information obtained when the test evaluation form in Appendix C is completed should be helpful in selecting those test instruments that are most appropriate for local use. It should also be useful in identifying specific aspects of tests that need to be modified. Guidelines for modifying tests and developing local norms are presented in chapter 7.

Administration of Tests

Once an appropriate test has been selected, procedures are needed to ensure that the instrument is administered in a manner that will yield valid assessment data. The examiner should be thoroughly familiar with the procedures for administering and scoring the test prior to assessing the child. The procedures for test administration described in the test manual must not be altered if the published test norms are to be used in interpreting results obtained from the instrument.

During the administration of tests, the examiner must be aware of variables in the context of the testing situation that may influence performance. When speech–language evaluations are conducted in a structured clinical environment rather than in a naturalistic setting, the language behavior observed may not be representative of the individual's true capabilities. Moreover, specific examiner characteristics may influence test performance.

> A Black, Navajo, or Chicano child before an adult white interviewing listener may demonstrate what may seem like extremely limited vocabulary, hesitations, uncoordinated or unstructured physical motion, a sense of disinterest and unease, which upon dismissal from that setting and return to another social situation of familiarity and one of less personal threat produces a very different complex of social and language interactions. (Bronstein, 1973, p. 694)

Individuals involved in the administration of speech and language tests must have an understanding of the child's culture and way of life. Without this background, one is likely to experience difficulty establishing rapport with the child. Moreover, an understanding of the child's culture is essential to ensure that cultural differences are distinguished from behaviors that are indicative of a disorder. Patterns of behavior that are common to members of a particular cultural group must not be viewed as deficiencies (Watson, Omark, Grouell, & Heller, 1981).

Another factor to consider in test administration is the child's background in taking tests. The child may have had no previous experience with tests and may not understand the purpose of testing. Moreover, the test may require the performance of behaviors that the child has never been asked to perform in any other context.

Formal testing should not be initiated until the child has been provided with the background necessary to respond appropriately to the tasks on the test. The child should be familiar with all aspects of the testing situation and must understand what is expected on the test. Preparing the child for the types of tasks included on the test will maximize the probability of valid test results.

Guidelines for Test Interpretation

Tests can serve a valuable function in the assessment of bilingual children with suspected communicative disorders if professionals are sensitive to the limitations of these measures and exercise caution in test interpretation. The following guidelines are recommended when using tests in the identification of communicatively handicapped bilingual children.

Test scores should not be used as the sole basis for identifying bilingual children with communicative disorders. A common practice in assessment is to determine a child's eligibility for special education services (e.g., speech–language remediation) based on how test scores compare to normative data.

As mentioned previously, test norms fail to consider differences among children in the amount and type of language exposure that they have had. Thus, there may not be any tests available that were standardized on an appropriate comparison group for the child being assessed.

When children achieve low scores on tests, it is important to examine the reason for their poor performance. Low scores on tests can result from lack of motivation, test anxiety, an inability to understand the test instructions, and a variety of other factors. Assessment personnel must be sensitive to individual differences that may account for specific problems observed in the testing situation.

To identify the specific factors contributing to a child's poor performance on a test, the specific types of errors produced and the consistency of these errors should be examined. Errors that are not typical of other children in the community with similar language backgrounds should be viewed as evidence of a possible disorder. Educational decisions, however, should never be based solely on the results of a single test instrument. Tests results should always be compared with data obtained from other measures.

The contexts in which the child has had opportunities to use each language need to be considered in the analysis of responses produced on tests. A Japanese-dominant student in a kindergarten classroom where only English is used will acquire only English language concepts in that setting. Thus, lexical items first experienced by the child in the school setting (e.g., words such as *chalk, bulletin board,* and *recess*) may be known only in English. The child's inability to name these items in Japanese is not an indication of a communicative disorder because the individual has had no experience with these concepts in Japanese. Thus, the child's test performance in each language must be evaluated in relation to the amount and type of language exposure experienced in various contexts.

The extent to which test performance is influenced by cultural and environmental factors unique to the individual being assessed needs to be explored (see chap. 4). Two children from the same cultural background may differ in the extent to which they have been exposed to the customs, values, and beliefs of that culture. Moreover, each child interacts with the environment in unique ways. Assessment personnel must view each child as a unique individual in the interpretation of test data. Reviewing the test results with the child's parents can often provide information about cultural and environmental factors that may have affected the child's performance on the test.

Test results should always be used in conjunction with information obtained from natural communication samples. Tests provide indications of *possible* problems that the child may be experiencing during natural communication activities. Some children may perform poorly on structured tests, however, because of difficulties in responding to the test format. Hence, structures that cause the individual no difficulty during natural speaking activities may be produced in error on tests. When test results suggest the presence of a disorder, further assessment is needed to determine if the problem is also evident in natural speaking contexts.

The analysis of natural communication samples is also necessary so that problems in the child's functional use of language can be identified. A child should be considered to have a communicative disorder only if evidence of a deficit is found during conversational speech. Techniques that can be used to collect natural communication samples are described in the next chapter.

Chapter 6

Alternatives to Standardized Language Tests

If bilingual children are to be assessed in a nondiscriminatory manner, valid and reliable assessment instruments must be used. At present, no comprehensive system for assessing communicative disorders is available for children who speak a language other than English (Mercer, 1983). Standardized tests have been criticized because there appear to be "few, if any standardized measures that can provide a completely valid and nonbiased evaluation of handicapping conditions for linguistically and culturally diverse populations" (Taylor & Payne, 1983, pp. 9–10). The challenge to test developers was described by Vaughn-Cooke (1983):

> It is not an overstatement to say that a crisis exists in the area of assessment for non-mainstream speakers. Researchers, clinicians, and test developers must intensify their efforts to overcome this crisis and meet the needs of diagnosticians. Diagnosticians do not need more evaluations of the assessment problem, nor do they need more "interim" solutions. They need valid, reliable assessment tools. (p. 33)

The task of appropriately identifying bilingual children with communicative disorders is especially difficult in school districts serving children from a variety of language backgrounds. A small school district near San Diego, California, for example, has 19 different language groups represented within its student population. Most of those languages are not spoken by any of the teachers or paraprofessionals employed by the school district. When standardized tests are unavailable or inadequate for use with the local population, assessment personnel have to rely on other assessment strategies. This chapter provides a description of various alternatives to standardized tests that can be used in assessing the oral communication skills of bilingual children with suspected handicaps.

USE OF NATURAL COMMUNICATION SAMPLES

The analysis of samples of the child's natural communication can provide valuable information in the assessment of culturally and linguistically different children (Leonard & Weiss, 1983; Prutting, 1983). The effective use of natural communication samples requires that one have an understanding of normal communication development.

Information on developmental sequences is not available for many of the minority languages and dialects spoken in this country. Without such information, some researchers have argued that language sample analyses cannot provide sufficient information to judge the normalcy of the culturally different child's language.

> Language sample analyses cannot provide some of the critical information required to make a diagnosis regarding the normalcy of a child's language. For this reason they must be used in conjunction with appropriate standardized tests which are generally not available for non-mainstream speakers. Leonard, Prutting, Perozzi, and Berkley (1978) noted, quite correctly, that such tests serve at least one valuable purpose: "They separate the impaired language user from the normal language user" (p. 373). The first step, then, in the assessment process is to administer a norm-referenced test which can separate, validly and reliably, normal language from disordered language. Language sample analyses cannot accomplish this goal. (Vaughn-Cooke, 1983, p. 31)

It is our viewpoint, however, that natural language samples do, in fact, make it possible to distinguish normal language from disordered language if the child's communicative behavior is compared in a systematic manner to that of other children in the local community who have had similar cultural and linguistic experiences. Thus, one must become familiar with the local dialect and the language used in the school curriculum. Systematic observations of communicative interactions among nonhandicapped bilingual children are necessary so that normal behaviors can be distinguished from those that characterize the speech of children with communicative disorders. Interviews with adult speakers of the local dialect can be helpful in identifying cultural norms governing how children are expected to interact with others in various speaking contexts (see chap. 4).

The use of natural communication samples provides an opportunity to assess the child's behavior in real life settings where there is a need to communicate (Prutting, 1983). When communication is assessed in context, both verbal and nonverbal aspects of the child's behavior can be examined. It is recommended that the assessment process begin with informal observations of the child's behavior during communicative interactions with others in the environment. The classroom, playground, and the school cafeteria are among the settings where such observations can be made. What will be seen is the ebb and flow of conversation in a variety of communicative contexts. In contrast to formal testing procedures which focus only on the behavior of the speaker, the assessment of communication in context allows one to examine an individual's communication in terms of its effect on the behavior of the listener.

A speech–language pathologist who does not speak the child's language cannot assess what is being said without assistance from an interpreter. Even without knowing the child's language, however, it is possible to begin collecting information on the child's patterns of interaction with others in the environment. By observing the effect of the child's communication on the actions of the listener, clues are provided about what is happening during the interaction. Does the listener respond verbally, perform an action following a statement, or does the listener simply pay no attention to what is being said? Perhaps the listener will look quizzical, frown, stare at the speaker, or walk away. The observer needs to be familiar with the discourse rules and nonverbal behaviors that characterize interactions within the child's culture so that the appropriateness of these behaviors can be judged.

Some nonverbal behaviors are relatively universal (Ekman & Friesen, 1975, 1978) while others can still be understood across cultures (Eibl-Eibesfeldt, 1975; Omark & Watson, 1983a). When a child does not respond or appears separated from peers who speak the same language, there is reason for concern (Bates, 1976; Omark, 1981b). Even at the preschool level, normal children limit their interactions with communicatively handicapped peers (Erickson & Omark, 1980). Observing the facial expressions, gestures, and actions of the listener can provide relevant information about the abilities of the speaker.

As observations are made in natural speaking contexts, one should note the manner in which the child initiates interactions and how the child responds when interactions are initiated by others. Examples of behavioral observations that may be indicative of communicative disorders include the following:

1. Child rarely initiates verbal interactions with peers;
2. Peers rarely initiate verbal interactions with the child;
3. Child does not respond verbally when verbal interactions are initiated by peers;
4. Child's communication has little or no effect on the actions of peers;
5. Child does not engage in dialogue with peers;
6. Child generally uses gestures rather than speech to communicate;
7. Facial expressions, eye contact, and/or other nonverbal aspects of the child's communication are culturally inappropriate;
8. Facial expressions and/or actions of peers indicate that they may be having difficulty understanding the child's communication.

Collecting a Representative Communication Sample

In addition to observing the child informally in various speaking contexts, a representative communication sample should be audiotaped or videotaped so that the child's productive use of language can be assessed. The goal is to obtain a sample that is a valid and reliable measure of the child's communicative capabilities.

Interactors

The quantity and quality of the child's speech may vary depending on who is involved in the interaction. Thus, interactions between the child and the speech–language pathologist may yield data different from those obtained during interactions with peers or family members.

When an adult interviewer (e.g., speech–language pathologist) interacts with the child, an interest should be shown in what the child is saying, and the interviewer should be nondirective. A sample consisting entirely of responses to questions presented by the interviewer is not likely to be representative of the child's performance capabilities. The interviewer must listen to the child and must adapt to the child's level of development during the interaction (Miller, 1981).

Context and Materials

The sample should be collected in contexts where the child uses language functionally for communicative purposes. If sampling is conducted in a clinical environment, a context should be established that is conducive to natural communication. The collection of communication samples during interactions in which blocks, dolls, toy cars, and other materials are available is often effective in eliciting spontaneous speech from young children.

Prutting (1983) has recommended that two communicative settings be used in collecting the sample—this should be viewed as an absolute minimum. Communication must be observed as language is used for a variety of speaking purposes.

Sample Size

It is recommended that a minimum of 30 minutes of conversation be recorded for analysis purposes. Children 2 years of age and older generally produce between 100 and 200 utterances in a 30-minute sample (Miller, 1981). Some researchers maintain that a minimum of 100 utterances be obtained (Tyack & Gottsleben, 1974; Prutting, 1983) while others recommend 200 or more (Muma, 1978). The number of utterances needed to obtain a representative sample varies depending on how the child responds in the particular contexts where communication is sampled. Thus, the analysis of the initial 30-minute sample may lead to questions that can be answered only by further sampling of the child's oral communication.

Recording the Sample

As mentioned earlier, the sample should be either audiotaped or videotaped. If the sample is audiotaped, relevant contextual information may be missed. Therefore, it is recommended that notes be taken on what is happening during the interaction. These contextual notes are necessary to examine the contextual appropriateness of the child's utterances.

Transcription and Analysis of the Sample

The transcription of the sample should include the consecutive recording of all utterances produced by the child and others involved in the communicative interaction. When a bilingual speech–language pathologist is not available, it is recommended that two native speakers of the child's language make independent transcriptions of the sample. The transcriptions should be compared so that discrepancies can be resolved. The speech–language pathologist should then discuss each utterance with the individual who transcribed the sample and with one or more other speakers of the language to identify specific problems experienced by the child. A search for someone in the community who has expertise in the linguistic structure of the child's language (e.g., a professor of foreign languages or linguistics who is a native speaker) is well worth the effort.

A form such as that shown in Table 2 can be used to record the information obtained from those involved in the review of the communication sample. The procedure for completing the four sections of this form is as follows:

1. *Transcription.* Transcribe the child's utterances and those of the communicative partner. Phonological errors may be recorded directly above the words pronounced incorrectly. Relevant contextual information should be recorded in parentheses.
2. *Structure.* Record errors in syntax and morphology for each utterance that is ungrammatical within the child's dialect.
3. *Function.* Record the specific communicative function served by each utterance.
4. *Comments.* Record comments that have relevance in assessing the individual's effectiveness as a communicator. Comments relating to vocabulary use, appropriateness of responses, and the effect of the child's communication on the behavior of the listener may be recorded.

Assessment of Language Function

A child's ability to communicate effectively cannot be assessed by studying utterances produced in isolation. As an example, consider the utterance, "It's cold in here." Without contextual information, the communicative intent of this utterance cannot be determined (Walters, 1981). Thus, one must have information about the topic of discussion, situation in which the utterance is produced, and so forth, to evaluate a child's communicative competence.

The pragmatics of language, the study of the speaker's functional use of language in context, has been a major area of interest among researchers during the past decade (Bates, 1976; Briere, 1972; Sridhar, 1981; Walters, 1981). When a pragmatic framework is used in assessment, communicative

TABLE 2.
Sample Transcript Showing Interactions Between Child and Peer

Child's Name: Sample Transcribed By:

Birthdate: Total Number of Utterances:

Date of Evaluation:

Key:
C = Child being evaluated
P = Peer

Language Sample Transcription		Structure	Function	Comments
1.	**C:** Where is the ball?	Omission of article *the* before *ball*.	Request for information	
	P: There it is. (pointed to ball)			
2.	**C:** Get it.		Request for action	
	P: I don't want to.			
3.	**C:** Me like that car. (pointed to truck)	Substitution of pronoun *me* for *I*.	Statement of information	Referred to *truck* as *car*.
	P: What car? (kicked the ball)			Peer appeared not to understand what child was referring to.
4.	**C:** Don't do that!		Statement of protest	

effectiveness is examined by studying interactions between a speaker and a listener in a social context.

Observing Speech Acts

When communication is assessed in context, observations are made of the child's performance of basic units of meaningful communication referred to as *speech acts* (Austin, 1962). Greetings ("Hello!"), warnings ("Don't go there!"), and statements of information ("I found five cents") are all examples of speech acts. Searle (1969) proposed that speech acts generally are "made possible by and performed in accordance with certain rules for the use of linguistic elements" (p. 16). The rules governing the performance of speech acts are established by the conventions of society (Lucas, 1980). Therefore, one must be familiar with cultural differences in how speech acts are performed when culturally and linguistically different children are assessed.

The manner in which speech acts are performed varies with the context in which the speaker is observed. Labov (1971) found that individual speakers demonstrate shifts in their communication style under different sociolinguistic conditions. The formality of the situation, discourse topic, and role relationship among participants in the interaction influence one's communicative behavior. An individual, for example, may switch from a neighborhood dialect to a more standard form of speech in an environment where the standard dialect is more appropriate (Halliday, 1978).

Numerous taxonomies of speech acts and language functions can be used to assess children's communicative competence. Dore (1975) developed a taxonomy of nine speech acts observed in the one-word utterances of young children: labeling, repeating, answering, requesting answer, requesting action, calling, greeting, protesting, and practicing. A more elaborate scheme for categorizing the conversational acts produced in the speech of preschoolers has also been developed by Dore (1978).

Seven basic functions observed in the language of children before 2 years of age were described by Halliday (1975).

1. *Instrumental* ("I want!")—Use of language to satisfy the child's material needs;
2. *Regulatory* ("Do as I tell you")—Use of language to regulate the behaviors of others;
3. *Interactional* ("Me and you")—Use of language to establish or maintain interaction with the listener;
4. *Personal* ("Here I come")—Use of language to express personal identity;
5. *Heuristic* ("Tell me why")—Use of language to explore the environment and learn new things;
6. *Imaginative* ("Let's pretend")—Use of language to create an imaginary reality;
7. *Informative* ("I've got something to tell you")—Use of language to communicate new information to the listener.

Children eventually learn to combine these functions as their experiences in the use of language broaden and as they learn more about the world around them.

Tough (1977) described four language functions observed in the speech of children 3 years of age and older:

1. *Directive*—Use of language to direct the actions and operations of self and others;
2. *Interpretive*—Use of language to communicate the meaning of events;
3. *Projective*—Use of language to relate information that is not tied to immediate experiences (e.g., predicting, projecting into the experiences of others, imagining);
4. *Relational*—Use of language to establish and maintain relationships.

Familiarity with the various taxonomies that have been developed for classifying speech acts and language functions is helpful when assessing the pragmatic aspects of the child's oral communication. These taxonomies have been described in detail by Chapman (1981). It is recommended that the following procedures be followed in the functional analysis of data obtained from the child's transcribed communication sample.

A taxonomy should be selected that is appropriate for the age and cultural background of the child. Published taxonomies should be reviewed by individuals who are familiar with the cultural norms of the local population and the discourse rules that govern interactions. Existing taxonomies may need to be modified or expanded for local use.

Each speech act should be categorized in terms of its specific communicative function. This information can be analyzed quantitatively. Thus, the percentage of speech acts that were statements of information, requests for action, and so forth, can be calculated to examine the extent to which the child uses language for specific purposes. Some utterances serve more than one function and, therefore, need to be assigned to multiple categories in the analysis.

The effect of each speech act on the behavior of the listener should be examined. This information is necessary to assess the child's effectiveness in using the language for specific purposes. When a request for action is made by the child, for example, does the listener respond by performning that action? Is the child able to initiate conversations with others and to maintain a topic over a series of utterances? Problems noted in the child's ability to convey communicative intents effectively should be noted.

Observational Communication Inventories

Information obtained from the analysis of the child's communication sample can be supplemented by observational data obtained as the child is observed by relevant others in the school and home environment. A variety of inventories have been developed that can be used by speech–language pathologists, classroom teachers, and others to record naturalistic observations of specific problems observed in the bilingual child's functional use of language (Erickson, 1981; Mattes, 1984; Omark, 1981b).

Bilingual Oral Language Development (BOLD), an oral language inventory developed by the authors for elementary school children, is presented in Table 3.* The form can be used to record observations of the child's performance in both the native language and English. A plus (+) should be recorded for each communicative behavior that is performed effectively; A minus (−) should be recorded for each communicative behavior in which a deficiency is noted. The behaviors listed on the inventory are described below.

1. *Comments on own actions.* The child comments on personal actions while these actions are taking place. Example: "I'm working fast."
2. *Comments on others' actions.* The child comments on actions of others in the environment. Example: "He broke the pencil."
3. *Describes experiences accurately.* The child is able to give an accurate description of personal experiences.
4. *Describes events sequentially.* The child describes a sequence of events in the order in which they occurred.
5. *Attends to the speaker.* The child allows communicative partners to speak and shows appropriate listening behavior.
6. *Follows directions.* The child follows directions presented in the classroom setting.
7. *Initiates interactions.* The child initiates conversations with classmates.
8. *Takes turns during conversation.* The child alternates appropriately as speaker and listener during conversations with peers.
9. *Maintains topic.* The child is able to maintain a topic of discussion over a series of utterances during interactions with peers.
10. *Answers questions.* The child gives appropriate responses to simple questions.
11. *Requests attention.* The child uses language to seek the attention of others.
12. *Requests information.* The child asks questions to obtain information about people, actions, events, etc.
13. *Requests action.* The child uses language to direct the actions of others.
14. *Requests clarification.* The child requests clarification when verbal statements made by others are not understood.
15. *Expresses needs.* The child uses language to inform others of personal needs.
16. *Expresses feelings.* The child uses language to express feelings such as joy, fear, and anger.
17. *Describes plans.* The child describes plans for events that will take place in the future.
18. *Supports viewpoints.* The child expresses personal opinions and is able to provide a logical rationale for those opinions.

*Table 3 may be reproduced for use as an assessment tool.

TABLE 3.
Sample Communication Skills Inventory for Bilingual Children

Bilingual Oral Language Development

Child's Name:
Birthdate:
Child's First Language:
Child's Second Language:

	Communicative Behavior	First Language	Second Language
1.	Comments on own actions	1. ________	1. ________
2.	Comments on others' actions	2. ________	2. ________
3.	Describes experiences accurately	3. ________	3. ________
4.	Describes events sequentially	4. ________	4. ________
5.	Attends to the speaker	5. ________	5. ________
6.	Follows directions	6. ________	6. ________
7.	Initiates interactions	7. ________	7. ________
8.	Takes turns during conversation	8. ________	8. ________
9.	Maintains topic	9. ________	9. ________
10.	Answers questions	10. ________	10. ________
11.	Requests attention	11. ________	11. ________
12.	Requests information	12. ________	12. ________
13.	Requests action	13. ________	13. ________
14.	Requests clarification	14. ________	14. ________
15.	Expresses needs	15. ________	15. ________
16.	Expresses feelings	16. ________	16. ________
17.	Describes plans	17. ________	17. ________
18.	Supports viewpoints	18. ________	18. ________
19.	Describes solutions	19. ________	19. ________
20.	Expresses imagination	20. ________	20. ________

From Mattes, L. J., & Omark, D. R. (1984) *Speech and Language Assessment for the Bilingual Handicapped.* San Diego: College-Hill Press.

19. *Describes solutions.* The child describes solutions for simple problem situations.
20. *Expresses imagination.* The child uses language to express imagination through drama, storytelling, puppet shows, etc.

It is recommended that the child's performance on the inventory be evaluated based on direct observations made by assessment personnel or based on information obtained from the classroom teacher and others in the school environment. The results should be shared with the child's parents to determine if similar problems have been observed in the home. By consulting with the classroom teacher, parents, and others, one can examine how the child's communication varies in different contexts. When both of the child's languages are examined, the results may be used to determine the language in which the child functions best.

When BOLD and other observational inventories are used in assessment, modifications should be made, as necessary, to meet the needs of the particular ethnic group being assessed. What is viewed as a problem by one ethnic group may be viewed as completely normal by another ethnic group. It is not uncommon, for example, to observe Vietnamese children who do not ask questions in the classroom setting (Wei, 1983).

Observational inventories of functional communication skills can also be used in classroom screening programs. Traditionally, problems observed in the child's production of particular linguistic structures have served as the basis for referrals to the speech–language pathologist. A study conducted by Damico and Oller (1980), however, revealed that classroom teachers who were taught to use pragmatic criteria as a basis for referral were correct significantly more often in their identification of language-disordered children than were teachers who were taught to use the more traditional syntactic and morphological criteria. The specific pragmatic features that teachers learned to use in making referrals were linguistic nonfluencies, revisions, delays before responding, nonspecific vocabulary, inappropriate responses, poor topic maintenance, and need for repetition. These pragmatic behaviors have also been found to be effective in identifying limited English proficient children with handicaps (Damico, Oller, & Storey, 1983). Referral to a speech–language pathologist, however, is appropriate only for those limited English children who demonstrate problems in the use of their dominant language.

The pragmatic criteria studied in the research described above have been incorporated into Spotting Language Problems (Damico & Oller, 1984), an instrument designed for use in the classroom setting. This screening tool includes a description of the pragmatic referral criteria and specific procedures for scoring. Spotting Language Problems has been used in screening bilingual student populations in public school settings.

Adaptive Behavior Inventories

Observational communication inventories can be used in conjunction with adaptive behavior measures to provide a more complete picture of the individual's functional capabilities. Measures of adaptive behavior are designed to ascertain the child's level of functioning in a variety of situations in the environment.

Two widely used measures with normative data on non-Anglo children are the Adaptive Behavior Scale (Grossman, 1973) and the Adaptive Behavior Inventory for Children (Mercer, 1979). Although both of these measures can provide useful information, the Adaptive Behavior Inventory for Children is a more culturally appropriate instrument for use in the assessment of children from minority backgrounds. This inventory is completed by the child's parents and is designed for use in assessing the adaptive behavior of children between 5 and 12 years of age. Anglos, Blacks, and Chicanos were equally represented in the standardization sample, and separate norms are provided for each group.

Adaptive behavior measures typically include items designed to examine the child's interactions with others in various types of real life situations. Moreover, items are included that relate directly to the child's functional use of communication. When observational communication inventories are used in conjunction with adaptive behavior measures, a detailed case history, and other assessment information, it is possible to identify the various environmental factors that are having an impact on behavior. Oral communication must be examined in terms of its relationship to other aspects of the child's functioning if appropriate educational programs are to be provided.

Assessing Language Structure

During the past decade, numerous methods have been developed to assess English-speaking children's level of linguistic structural development using natural communication samples (e.g., Crystal, Fletcher, & Garman, 1976; Lee, 1974; Tyack & Gottsleben, 1974). Few such methods, however, are available for use in assessing children who speak languages other than English. Moreover, research on the acquisition of many of the languages spoken in our schools has not been conducted.

Several procedures have become available for assessing the spontaneous language of Spanish-speaking children. Linares (1981) developed a procedure for computing Spanish-speaking children's mean length of utterance. This measure is computed based on an analysis of 100 consecutive utterances. An approach for measuring the Spanish speaker's mean length of utterance has also been developed by Garcia, Maez, and Gonzalez (1981).

The Developmental Assessment of Spanish Grammar (DASG) (Toronto, 1976) was designed for use in assessing the grammatical performance of children between 3 and 6 years, 11 months of age. The procedure is based on Developmental Sentence Scoring (DSS) (Lee, 1974). The grammatical structures assessed using Toronto's procedure include (1) indefinite pronouns and noun modifiers, (2) personal pronouns, (3) primary verbs, (4) secondary verbs, (5) conjunctions, and (6) interrogatives. Normative data obtained on 128 Spanish-speaking children are provided. A major limitation of this procedure is that it is time-consuming and only a limited number of grammatical structures are assessed.

Developing procedures for recording, categorizing, and analyzing information obtained from natural communication samples is no simple task when speech–language pathologists are not available who speak the child's language. The first step in the process is to become familiar with the structure of the child's language. The following strategies can be used for this purpose.

1. Interview several fluent speakers of the child's language to find out as much as possible about that language and how it is used in the local community.
2. Review published research on language acquisition that includes information about the child's language.
3. Review publications describing the linguistic structure of the child's language. Textbooks used in foreign language courses can be helpful in identifying the various structural components of the language that need to be examined.

A comprehensive structural analysis of the child's communication will provide important information about the nature and extent of specific deficits exhibited by the child. The results of this analysis can then be used to develop appropriate goals for intervention. An effort should be made to obtain the services of a speech–language pathologist who speaks the child's language if there are no bilingual speech–language pathologists available locally to analyze the sample. Bilingual individuals who are not specifically trained as speech–language pathologists may be able to provide assistance in reviewing the individual utterances produced by the child. Monolingual speech–language pathologists should *always* share the communication sample with more than one bilingual speaker so that differences of opinion can be considered as individual utterances are reviewed. By sharing the communication sample with various bilingual community members, local standards can be used in judging the structural adequacy of the child's utterances.

ELICITED LANGUAGE PRODUCTION TASKS

Following the collection of a natural communication sample, specific aspects of the child's language behavior may need to be examined in further detail. Elicited production procedures can be used for this purpose.

> The use of elicited production procedures is warranted when specific aspects of language are to be analyzed, when frequency of occurrence in naturalistic settings is limited, or if the usual situations do not afford detailed analysis of a specific language behavior. Where time is a factor these procedures can be quite productive in eliciting the behaviors required in a short period of time. (Miller, 1981, p. 139)

Structured Language Sampling

This procedure involves the presentation of stimuli designed to elicit productions of particular communicative behaviors. To elicit production of the preposition *under*, for example, the examiner might present a picture showing a dog *under* a table and ask "Where is the dog?" Structured language sampling techniques can be used to measure the child's comprehension and production of particular language structures in a variety of sentence contexts and under different types of stimulus conditions.

Structured language sampling techniques can also be used to elicit particular language functions. The tasks employed, however, must establish conditions in which meaningful communication is produced or the results may not reflect the child's actual use of language in natural speaking contexts.

When structured language sampling techniques are used, the procedures should be adapted, as necessary, to meet the needs of the child. Tasks that have been effective when used in assessing Anglo children may not always be effective when used with children from other cultures.

Elicited Imitation

Elicited imitation tests use a "say what I say" approach in which the child's task is to repeat sentences after hearing them read by the examiner. The errors produced indicate possible problems that the child may be experiencing in natural speaking situations. Thus, a child who consistently omits pronouns, for example, may not be using pronouns correctly in spontaneous speech. Prutting and Connolly (1976) have warned that sentence imitation tasks may "underestimate, overestimate, or accurately describe the child's language performance" (p. 420). Thus, the results should always be used in conjunction with a natural communication sample.

The Elicited Language Analysis Procedure (Mattes, 1982b) provides a method for systematically evaluating responses on sentence imitation tasks in terms of both their syntactic and semantic relationships to the stimulus sentence presented. Overall grammatical acceptability, syntactic usage on specific grammatical forms, vocabulary usage, and response quality are the factors considered in scoring. This procedure can be useful in assessing children's control over grammar and their comprehension of verbal stimuli.

The Elicited Language Analysis Procedure is appropriate for children from any cultural or linguistic background. The stimulus sentences used in sentence imitation, however, must be constructed to reflect the structure of the language being assessed.

Criterion-Referenced Tests

Criterion-referenced tests can be used to assess the extent to which the child has mastered specific communication skills. These measures are designed to ascertain the child's level of performance in relation to a specific criterion.

The Comprehensive Inventory of Basic Skills (Brigance, 1983) includes criterion-referenced tasks designed to assess the child's performance in a variety of school-related skills. Listening and speaking are among the areas assessed. A Spanish adaptation of this inventory has also been developed (Brigance, 1984).

Mattes (1982a) developed a comprehensive inventory of criterion-referenced tasks for assessing the listening and speaking abilities of English-speaking children. Instructional activities are provided for each of the skills assessed. Many of the criterion-referenced tasks included in this inventory could be adapted quite easily for use in other languages.

Spanish Language Assessment Procedures (Mattes, 1984) is an inventory designed specifically for use in assessing the communication skills of Spanish-speaking children at the elementary school level. Criterion-referenced tests and naturalistic observation techniques are used to assess the structural and functional aspects of communication. Measures of articulation, language, voice, and fluency are included in the inventory.

USE OF STORY CONTEXTS IN ASSESSMENT

Short stories can be used in various ways to examine the child's communicative capabilities within meaningful contexts. Story retelling and the cloze procedure are examples of techniques in which short stories are used.

Story Retelling Tasks

Story retelling tasks are designed to assess the child's ability to retell a short story immediately after hearing it read by the examiner. An age-appropriate story relevant to the interests and cultural background of the child should be used. It is recommended that assessment begin with a story between 100 and 150 words in length when children between 5 and 8 years of age are assessed. Longer stories may be used in assessing older children. The retelling of the story should be audiotaped.

At the completion of the retelling, questions should be asked by the examiner to examine the child's comprehension of story content. These questions should be general (e.g., "Where did the story take place?") and should not provide the child with information that has not already been stated in the retelling of the story.

The audiotaped retelling of the story can be used to assess the child's effectiveness in describing events and organizing information into an appropriate sequence. Thus, the child's use of language to convey meaning can be analyzed. By using a graded series of passages, the child's comprehension and production can be assessed at varying levels of difficulty.

The administration of story retelling tasks to bilingual children in both languages provides information that is helpful in identifying the dominant language. A story retelling task is included in the Language Assessment Scales (DeAvila & Duncan, 1977), a language dominance measure, but the scoring procedure is based primarily on language structure rather than function. Both the structural and functional aspects of language should be examined when story retelling tasks are used in language dominance testing.

Cloze Procedure

The cloze procedure is a technique in which words are deleted from a passage at regular intervals, and the child's task is to supply the missing words. The procedure can be used to assess both oral language functioning and reading comprehension. When the cloze procedure is used in reading assessment, the child is asked to fill in the deleted words after reading a 250-word passage in which every 5th word is missing (Bormuth, 1968; Hittleman, 1978). Performance on cloze tests has been found to correlate significantly with performance on reading comprehension measures (Alexander, 1968; Bormuth, 1969; Page, 1977). The procedure has been used successfully with speakers of English, Japanese, Thai, Vietnamese, Swedish, and numerous other languages (Grundin, Courtney, Langer, Pehrrson, Robinson, & Sakamoto, 1978; Oller, Bowen, Dien, & Mason, 1972). Moreover, performance on cloze tests has proven to be effective in the assessment of second-language proficiency (Oller, 1979).

Oral Adaptation of the Cloze Procedure

An oral adaptation of the cloze test that can be used in assessing children's oral language proficiency is described below.

1. Developing the Cloze Test

   A. Select a complete story between 250 and 350 words in length. A published story or a story developed by a bilingual speaker from the local community may be used.
   B. Remove every 5th, 6th, or 7th word until 50 words are deleted. Do not selectively remove a particular type of word (e.g., prepositions).
   C. Do not remove the first word in a sentence or any proper noun—skip to the next word.
   D. Tape-record the story if more than one child is to be tested.

2. Presenting the Cloze Test

   A. Present several examples of what is expected by reading sentences with a word deleted and asking the child to supply that word.

      Example: "Mr. Lopez broke his ________ yesterday."

      The examiner should signal the spot where the word is missing by making a sound (e.g., clicking the tongue).
   B. Present the entire story to the child without any words deleted.
   C. Ask the child several general questions about the content of the story. If the child has difficulty answering these questions, present the story a second time.
   D. Begin the testing. Read to the point where the first word is deleted, signal the deletion (e.g., click the tongue), and then read to the end of that phrase or sentence.

E. Read the sentence a second time, but this time pause to allow the child to supply the missing word.
F. Continue this process until the end of the story.

Either an *exact* word method or an *approximate* word method can be used in scoring the cloze test. In the exact word method, the child's response must be identical to the word in the passage to receive credit. In the approximate word method, the child receives credit for any word that does not alter the author's intended meaning. The approximate word method will result in a higher score.

A qualitative analysis of individual responses can reveal specific deficiencies that may be reducing the child's communicative effectiveness. Each response that is *not* identical to the word that was deleted from the story should be examined carefully. Does the response fit grammatically within the sentence in which it was produced? Does the response maintain the meaning that the author of the passage intended to convey? Does the response result in a sentence that makes no sense at all? Use of the cloze procedure makes it possible to examine the interaction of the syntactic and semantic systems within a context that has meaning.

In the sense that the procedure involves an interaction between the child and a meaningful context, it can be viewed as a pragmatic measure (see Oller, 1979). Administration of the cloze procedure to a bilingual child in both languages allows for the assessment of language dominance within a contextual situation.

The oral cloze technique has been used to assess the language skills of native English speakers (Cracker, 1971; Nutter, 1974) and to assess the English language proficiency of second-language learners (Scholz, Hendricks, Spurling, Johnson, & Vandenburg, 1980; Stevenson, 1974). There currently is no published research on the use of the oral cloze technique to identify bilingual children with communicative disorders. Comments we have received from practitioners using this procedure, however, indicate that cloze tests have potential as a tool for the assessment of communicative disorders.

NONSTANDARDIZED ASSESSMENT TECHNIQUES AND HANDICAP IDENTIFICATION

This chapter has reviewed a variety of alternatives to norm-referenced language tests that can be used in the assessment of bilingual children with suspected communicative disorders. Although norm-referenced tests can be helpful in distinguishing normal from disordered language, they do not provide sufficient information to identify the specific areas in which remediation is needed.

> The very fact that standardized test results are in quantitative terms makes the progress from test to treatment problematic. A finding that a child performs below the tenth percentile on a given test does not provide an indication of the feature of language

> that should serve as the initial or subsequent focus of remediation. (Leonard et al., 1978, p. 373)

A child should not be considered to have a communicative disorder until the specific manifestations of that disorder have been identified in natural communication contexts. The child's communication should be analyzed both quantitatively and qualitatively, using a variety of assessment tools. The use of natural communication samples and other nonstandardized approaches to assessment provides the in-depth description of the child's communication system necessary to identify that child's specific needs.

Chapter 7

Modifying and Constructing Assessment Instruments

There is a need for local school districts to become involved in the development of valid and reliable assessment tools for use in the identification of bilingual children with communicative disorders. The local development of tests makes it possible to compare the child's performance with that of peers from the same environment (Toronto & Merrill, 1983). This chapter presents specific guidelines that can be used within school districts to develop instruments for assessing the bilingual child's speech and language functioning.

Each school has different needs and the instruments used in assessment must reflect those needs. The school described below is fictitious, but the problems are typical of those that have been experienced in many school settings throughout the nation:

> Ordinary Elementary School is located in a small farm community and serves 600 students from diverse cultural and linguistic backgrounds. Of these 600 students, 250 are monolingual English speakers. The remaining 350 students demonstrate at least minimal proficiency in one of the following languages:

Language Spoken	**Number of Students**
Spanish	200
Vietnamese	85
Arabic	27
Samoan	18
Chincsc (Mandarin)	14
Tagalog	6
	350

> Although several teachers and instructional aides speak Spanish, none of the other minority languages is spoken by anyone in the school setting. Bilingual instructional aides have assisted the speech–language pathologist in assessing Spanish-speaking children by using commercially

available Spanish assessment instruments. These tests, however, are all written in dialects different from that used in the local community.

The school currently has no tests available for bilingual speakers of languages other than Spanish. Speakers of Vietnamese, Arabic, Samoan, Chinese, and Tagalog have been referred for assessment but have not been tested. The speech–language pathologist is concerned about the problem.

What steps should be taken to improve testing procedures when schools are faced with a problem such as that described above? One alternative might be to use modified versions of existing tests or to translate English tests into other languages. Possibly new tests could be constructed for each of the languages spoken in the school setting. Some action has to be taken so that the referred students can be assessed.

ADAPTING EXISTING ASSESSMENT INSTRUMENTS FOR LOCAL USE

When published assessment instruments are inadequate to meet the needs of children in the local population, it is not always necessary to construct completely new tests. Published instruments can often be adapted in various ways to improve their validity for use in assessing a population different from that used in test standardization. Some instruments can be adapted more easily than others. Therefore, the selection of a test for local adaptation should always be preceded by a comprehensive review of factors such as the purpose of the instrument, procedures used in developing test content, and the manner in which individual test items are structured.

Using Translations of English Tests

The speech–language pathologist at Ordinary Elementary School, the school described in the case study, has had children referred from a variety of language backgrounds but does not have appropriate instruments for assessing these children. A common practice when faced with this problem is to translate English tests into the other languages in which testing is to be conducted. Examples of some of the problems that are likely to occur when English tests are translated into Spanish were described in chapter 5. Problems resulting from structural differences between languages are also apparent when tests are translated into languages such as Arabic, Chinese, or Vietnamese.

In contrast to English, Vietnamese words do not have prefixes or suffixes. Spoken Chinese languages (e.g., Mandarin), on the other hand, use a variety of prefixes and suffixes. The participle *bu*, for example is used as a prefix on verbs in Mandarin to negate the action of the verb (Tewksbury, 1948). These structural differences are among those that would not be considered if a translation of an English language test were used.

In some languages (e.g., Chinese, Vietnamese), words are pronounced using different tones to express different meanings. Two words may differ, for example, only in that one has a rising pitch on the vowel while the other has a falling pitch. The use of tones is an important aspect of language production that is not examined systematically if children are administered a literal translation of an English test.

The language tests that are easiest to translate are vocabulary measures in which knowledge of isolated words is assessed. Many English words, however, have no direct equivalent in languages such as Arabic, Chinese, Samoan, or Vietnamese and, therefore, cannot be translated. Moreover, some of the items are likely to be culturally inappropriate. Thus, efforts to develop literal translations of measures such as the Peabody Picture Vocabulary Test (Dunn & Dunn, 1981) may result in tests that are of questionable validity. The Peabody Picture Vocabulary Test is among the instruments that have been questioned in terms of their cultural appropriateness for children from minority backgrounds (Britton & Britton, 1981; Vaughn-Cooke, 1983).

The basic question that the speech–language pathologist must consider prior to selecting tests for translation is, "What type of information do I need to obtain?" Each test being considered for translation must be evaluated in terms of the extent to which a translation maintains the intended purpose of the test and provides valid information about the child's communicative capabilities.

It is important that the purpose and content of tests be reviewed by fluent speakers of the languages in which translations are to be developed. This review process will make it possible to identify specific problems that might result from translation. Will a translation of the test adequately measure the important structural components of the child's language? Will the translated test change the length of the stimulus words or sentences to such an extent that the original purpose of the test is defeated? These are among the questions that must be considered.

When literal translations of tests are used, changes are observed in grammatical structure, word and sentence length, stress patterns, and so forth. Some test items may need to be eliminated while others may need to be modified. It is also necessary, in most cases, to add additional items to the test so that the instrument reflects the important structural components of the child's language.

Modifying Test Content

The previous section discussed the need for test modifications when tests are translated into other languages. The need for test modifications, however, is not limited to situations in which tests are translated. Whenever the cultural and/or linguistic background of the child being assessed is different from that of the children in the test standardization sample, there may be a need for changes in the test content.

Tests standardized on Anglo children are often used to assess the English language proficiency of children from bilingual backgrounds (Mattes, 1982c). A non-Anglo, bilingual child who is able to communicate effectively in English may perform poorly on these measures because of culturally inappropriate test items or items that do not reflect the dialect of the local community. The elimination or modification of these inappropriate items can improve the validity of the instrument as a measure of spoken language proficiency for the local population. Vaughn-Cooke (1983) has emphasized that adequate modifications of traditional tests can be developed only if "test modifiers obtain a thorough knowledge of non-mainstream dialects before initiating revisions" (p. 31).

When a test designed for speakers of a language other than English is used, modifications may be necessary so that the test content reflects the experiences of the local bilingual population. The language content of a Spanish vocabulary test standardized on Mexican American children in California, for example, generally will need to be modified when used in assessing Puerto Rican children in New York. Differences in cultural experiences must also be considered in the review of test content.

Speech–language pathologists need to work with fluent speakers of the local dialect in the development of appropriate test modifications. Bilingual education teachers, bilingual instructional aides, and others may participate in this process.

Prior to using any published test instrument to assess bilingual children with suspected communicative disorders, it is recommended that the instrument be administered to a small randomly selected sample of students. The test instrument and the results of the field-testing should then be shared with several fluent speakers of the local dialect so that they can suggest areas in which the content of the test needs to be modified. These individuals must understand the purpose of each test item so that they can evaluate the test content effectively. Based on the information obtained, test items should be added, deleted, and/or modified to represent more adequately the cultural and linguistic experiences of children in the local population. New and modified test items should be field-tested prior to including them in the test instrument.

One should not be disturbed by the prospect of modifying a test. Modifications designed to improve the cultural and linguistic appropriateness of test items will result in a product that has greater validity for use in the identification of children with communicative disorders. Thus, the instrument will be more useful in the local school district.

There is nothing illegal about modifying the content of test items for local use. One must not, however, engage in activities such as changing the title of the test, claiming to be the author, or reproducing copies that are sold for profit. Moreover, it is recommended that the authors of the test be informed of the modifications that have been made so that they can offer their input and suggestions.

When modifications are made in standardized tests, the original normative data are nullified and must never be used in test interpretation. Moreover, the reliability and validity of the instrument will have to be reassessed.

Procedures for norming tests and establishing reliability and validity are described later in this chapter.

The development of test norms is *not* an absolute necessity for the test to serve a useful diagnostic function. An analysis of performance on individual test items may provide an indication of specific abnormalities in the child's comprehension and/or use of the spoken language. These behaviors can then be examined in further detail based on data obtained from natural communication samples and various informal language measures. Those communicative behaviors that are rarely observed among other children in the community who come from the same culture and language background should be viewed as evidence of a possible communicative disorder.

DEVELOPING NEW ASSESSMENT INSTRUMENTS AT THE LOCAL LEVEL

The adaptation of existing tests for use in other languages is often difficult because of the structural differences that exist between languages. As indicated earlier, translations of tests are often inappropriate because they do not reflect the structure of the language being assessed. When tests are not available in the child's language, there is often no alternative other than to develop new assessment instruments at the local level.

The development of tests in languages other than English requires that the speech–language pathologist work closely with bilingual individuals from the local community. The assistance of these bilingual consultants is necessary so that tests can be developed that reflect the structure of the language as it is used by the local student population.

Developing Articulation Measures

The construction of articulation tests requires that one become familiar with the phonological system of the language in which the test is to be developed. The phonemes that occur in each of the 15 most common minority languages in the United States are presented in Appendix D. Although languages differ in their phonological structure, a core inventory of phonemes exists that is common to most of the major languages of the world (see Ruhlen, 1976). The alphabet of the International Phonetic Association is used below to represent the 10 consonant phonemes in this core inventory:

1. Stops: p, b, t, d, k, g
2. Nasals: m, n
3. Glides: w, j

The phonemes in the core inventory are learned early by young children. Japanese-speaking children have been found to demonstrate correct production of phonemes in the core inventory by age 3 (Yasuda, 1970). Developmental data reported by Prather, Hedrick, and Kern (1975) for English speakers indicate that children 3 years of age generally are able to produce these sounds correctly in the initial and final position of words. Most consonants that are not in the core inventory, however, are acquired after the child's third birthday. In the absence of published norms for articulation development in most minority languages, a child's performance should always be compared to that of peers in the local community who have had similar cultural and linguistic experiences.

Articulation tests should be designed to assess children's production of phonemes in a variety of contexts. Pictures and objects can be used to elicit the child's production of words containing the various phonemes of the language. Stimulus materials (e.g., words used to test phonemes) should be reviewed by native speakers of the language and field-tested prior to including them in the instrument.

Instruments developed for use in articulation assessment should provide sufficient information to examine the child's use of specific phonological processes. The phonological processes that characterize the speech of English-speaking children with articulation disorders have been described in the literature (Compton, 1970; Hodson & Paden, 1983; Laila Khan, 1982). Based on a review of published studies, Laila Khan (1982) found that the most frequently noted processes were the following:

1. Affrication
2. Assimilation
3. Cluster reduction
4. Final consonant deletion
5. Coalescence
6. Final consonant devoicing
7. Fronting and backing
8. Gliding
9. Glottal replacement
10. Metathesis
11. Prevocalic voicing
12. Reduplication of syllables
13. Stopping
14. Vocalization
15. Deletion of weak syllables
16. Idiosyncratic processes

The above list of phonological processes may need to be modified somewhat when articulation tests are constructed in languages other than English. Many of the above processes, however, may be observed among minority language speakers with articulation disorders. Spanish-speaking children with highly unintelligible speech, for example, have been found to use phonological processes that have also been observed among English-speaking children (Hodson, Diamond, Meza, & Cornejo, 1983).

Locally developed articulation tests should be field-tested to assess the adequacy of the test instructions, stimulus materials, and test items. Modifications should be made based on the information obtained. Local norms can be developed by administering the test to various age groups and determining the percentage of children who produce each phoneme correctly in the various contexts assessed.

The test results should be compared to information obtained from other measures to determine the diagnostic usefulness of the instrument. It is especially important to examine the extent to which the instrument is effective in identifying the specific articulation problems that are experienced by children in conversational speech.

Developing Standardized Language Tests

Bilingual children with communicative disorders can be identified without standardized tests by obtaining a representative natural communication sample and comparing the child's performance with that of bilingual peers in the local community. Many school districts, however, require that standardized tests be used in assessment. If standardized tests are to be used, instruments must be available that yield valid and reliable results when administered to children in the local population. When such instruments do not exist, it becomes necessary for tests to be developed at the local level.

The development of standardized tests is most appropriate in school settings where a large number of students need to be assessed. The task of developing norms can be accomplished efficiently and effectively if a team approach is used in which speech–language pathologists work closely with bilingual educators, administrators, curriculum specialists, and others. The easiest approach is to standardize tests on a regional basis by working with other districts.

It is beyond the scope of this book to provide a detailed description of the procedures involved in standardizing tests and developing norms. The guidelines that follow, however, should be helpful in developing an appropriate test for local use.

Developing Objectives

Test construction must begin with careful planning. The first objective is to develop specific objectives for the test and to define the target population that will be tested using the instrument. What should the test be designed to measure? What age groups will be tested using the instrument? How will the results be used? These questions should be answered before any test items are constructed.

Developing Test Content

The speech–language pathologist should develop a pool of test items by working with native speakers of the language in which the test is being constructed. The item pool should then be submitted to a team of professionals and local community members for review. It is recommended that the team include someone with experience in statistical analysis procedures. Those items that are judged by the reviewers to be poorly constructed or culturally and/or linguistically inappropriate should be discarded.

Field-Testing the Instrument

The field-test version of the instrument should be administered to at least 25 children at each age or grade level for which the test is designed (Toronto & Merrill, 1983). Some of the items will, most likely, prove to be unsuitable and need to be discarded following field-testing. Therefore, the field-test version of the instrument should contain more items than are actually needed for the test.

An analysis of the students' performance on individual test items (i.e., item analysis) should be conducted to determine which items are suitable and which items need to be eliminated or modified. The average percentage of children passing a test item should be about 50%. Items generally are considered acceptable when the percentage of students responding correctly is between 15 and 85% (Anastasi, 1976).

Following the analysis of the data obtained during field testing, any necessary modifications should be made in the test items and the directions. These modifications should be field-tested prior to norming the test.

Developing Local Norms

When local norms are developed, the characteristics of the normative sample must reflect the characteristics of the individual students who will be assessed using the test instrument. Specific criteria should be established for the selection of children for the normative sample. Language dialect, socioeconomic level, length of residency in the United States, and a variety of other variables should be considered (see Gamez-Huebner, Watson, & Omark, 1984).

It is generally not appropriate to select a totally random sample of all speakers of a particular language when standardizing a test. If, for example, a test has been designed for use in assessing Spanish-dominant children who have been classified as limited English proficient, it is inappropriate for the sample to include English-dominant children who speak only a few words of Spanish. It must not be assumed that all children from a particular language background are *the same* when selecting children for the normative sample.

If normative data are to be useful, it is important that a large sample of students be tested. School district personnel with expertise in statistical analysis procedures should be consulted to ensure that adequate sampling procedures are used in norming the test. When the population of target students in the local school district is small, more than one school district should participate in collecting test data.

Once the testing has been completed, the children in the sample should be divided into groups by chronological age for data analysis purposes. Two basic measures that need to be computed for each group are the mean test score and the standard deviation. The measurement of performance in terms of how many standard deviations a child scores above or below the mean is often used as the basis for determining a child's eligibility for a special education program. A school district, for example, may require that a child score 1.5 standard deviations below the mean to qualify for enrollment in a remedial speech–language program. Children who score 1.5 standard deviations below the mean may need the services of a speech–language pathologist, but it is also possible that the normative data for the test are not normally distributed. Thus, the actual curve may over- or underestimate the number of children with handicaps (Omark & Watson, 1983a).

Measuring Test Reliability and Validity

Both test reliability (i.e., the consistency with which the test yields the same results) and validity (i.e., the extent to which the test measures what it was designed to measure) need to be examined. The specific procedures that will be used to assess the reliability and validity of the instrument should be planned prior to test standardization.

The most important reliability measure is test–retest reliability. This measure is computed by testing a group of children and then testing them a short time later (e.g., within 2 weeks) on the same measure. A test is considered highly reliable if children's scores on the second administration of the test are about the same as the scores obtained during the initial testing. Test–retest reliability can be computed using the Spearman rank order correlation or the Pearson product–moment correlation. The Spearman rank order correlation is easier to compute, but the Pearson product–moment correlation is considered a better measure. A reliability coefficient of .80 or higher generally is accepted as the minimum criterion for an assessment instrument that is to be used with individual children (Newcomer & Hammill, 1982; Watson, Omark, Grouell, & Heller, 1981).

Validity is always specific to some particular use of the test (Gronlund, 1981). The measurement of test validity must not be limited to an examination of the content of the instrument. The actual use of the instrument as an assessment tool also must be examined. A test that is designed for use in identifying bilingual children with communicative disorders, for example, must be validated specifically for this purpose.

Tests used to identify children with communicative disorders must provide results that distinguish between children known to have communication deficits and children who communicate well verbally. One approach used in the measurement of validity is to compare the test performance of a group of normal children with the test performance of a group of children known to have communicative disorders. Statistically significant differences should be observed between groups if the test is valid for its intended purpose.

Another approach often used in assessing validity is to examine the relationship between performance on the test and performance on other measures. For example, one could examine the extent to which children's scores on the test correlate with their scores on other language tests. One could also study the relationship between scores on the test and teachers' ratings of children's language proficiency. If the correlation is low, the usefulness of the test must be questioned.

It is also possible to examine validity by comparing children's performance on the test with their performance during natural communication activities. Do the specific errors produced by children on the test also occur in their spontaneous speech? Tests used in assessment should provide information that reflects children's performance capabilities in natural speaking contexts.

The measurement of reliability and validity should not be neglected when new tests are constructed or when existing tests are modified. Professionals (e.g., assessment specialists, statisticians) who are knowledgeable about methods for assessing reliability and validity should be consulted to ensure that appropriate procedures are used to obtain these measures. A comprehensive review of language test manuals can be helpful in the development of such procedures. The Test of Language Development (Newcomer & Hammill, 1982) and the Peabody Picture Vocabulary Test (Dunn & Dunn, 1982), for example, both include a discussion of the various types of reliability and validity and a description of the procedures used to obtain these measures.

Use of Test Scores

Test scores derived from standardized tests should always be used in conjunction with supportive data, even when the test in normed locally. Prior to placing a bilingual child into a program for children with communicative disorders, the specific nature of the disorder needs to be identified. Test scores alone do not provide this information. Leonard et al. (1978) emphasized that

> It is difficult to defend speech–language pathologists' roles in language assessment if assessment consists merely of derived scores, language ages, or percentiles. Presumably, the reason why speech–language pathologists are best equipped to assess the communication skills of language-impaired children is that we have also been trained in matters involving children's development and use of behaviors important to communication. It is this training that is called on in the adoption of nonstandardized measures; and it is this training that we need to apply if we are to serve language-impaired children adequately, and demonstrate that we have an important service to offer in the area of language assessment. (pp. 375–376)

Developing Nonstandardized Language Measures

Criterion-referenced tasks and a variety of other nonstandardized approaches to assessment were described in chapter 6. Leonard et al. (1978) emphasized that "the use of nonstandardized measures is essential in gaining sufficient information about the child's linguistic system in order to devise effective intervention strategies" (p. 371). A criterion-referenced communication skills inventory can be developed locally in which nonstandardized measures are used to examine specific structural and functional aspects of the child's communication. The information obtained for this inventory can be used to identify children with communicative disorders and to plan individualized programs.

Although the use of criterion-referenced instruments has been recommended as an alternative to standardized tests (Bailey & Harbin, 1980; Duffey et al., 1981), the criterion-referenced approach has not been without criticism. One of the major problems in using this approach in the assessment of minority children is that "there is no valid developmental sequence which can be used to specify which linguistic behaviors should be selected as a goal for a particular child" (Vaughn-Cooke, 1983, p. 31). Without this developmental information, one has no basis for establishing the criteria that will be used to evaluate children's performance on these measures.

The communicative capabilities of normal children at different grade levels in the school setting need to be examined so that a communication skills inventory can be developed that is effective in distinguishing normal children from children who demonstrate communicative disorders. Systematic observations of children's communicative behavior and an analysis of the oral language competencies necessary for children to function effectively in the classroom can provide the information needed to develop the inventory.

Information about normal children's communicative capabilities can also be obtained by interviewing classroom teachers and bilingual community members. A kindergarten teacher in a bilingual education classroom, for example, should be able to provide the speech–language pathologist with information about the types of communicative behaviors that typically are observed among kindergarten children. Cultural differences in how the language is used need to be considered in selecting the specific communicative behaviors that are included in the inventory.

Community members who speak the local dialect can provide valuable assistance to speech–language pathologists in the construction of a communication skills inventory. When local bilingual speakers work with the speech–language pathologist, an inventory can be constructed that is relevant to the interests and cultural experiences of children in the local community. Short stories used on tasks designed to assess the child's ability to retell stories in sequence, for example, can be developed by asking a local community member to tell a familiar folktale or describe a culturally familiar event. Tending sheep, going to the market, preparing a meal, or building a boat are among the events that could be described. The language dialect will be appropriate, and the content will be meaningful to children from the local population.

Behaviors on the communication skills inventory that occur frequently in natural speaking contexts generally can be evaluated based on systematic observations of the child during interactions with peers. Performance on some of the skills, however, may need to be assessed using criterion-referenced elicited production tasks. An example of an elicited production task designed for use in assessing the child's ability to name basic shapes is presented below.

Skill:

Child names shapes.

Procedure:

Pictures of a *circle, square, rectangle,* and *triangle* are placed in front of the child. The examiner points to each picture and asks, "What shape is this?"

Mastery Criterion:
The child names all four shapes correctly.

Tasks can also be developed to elicit the use of language for specific functions:

Skill:
Child requests objects.

Procedure:
The child is presented with a situation in which a task must be completed, but an object necessary for completion of the task is not available.

Example: The child is asked to draw a picture. A piece of paper is placed in front of the child but the child is not given anything to write with. Therefore, the child must make a request for something to write with.

Mastery Criterion:
The child is observed to request the missing object.

A review of published communication skills inventories should be helpful in the development of assesment strategies for local use. Criterion-referenced procedures that can be used to elicit speech acts in a structured setting with conversational dialogue were described by Lucas (1980) for the eight speech acts included in the Behavioral Inventory of Speech Act Performances. The criterion-referenced approach used in Spanish Language Assessment Procedures (Mattes, 1984) can also serve as a model for locally developed inventories.

The specific tasks developed for use in assessment should be field-tested on normal children prior to using them in the assessment of children with suspected handicaps. One can begin by administering a battery of tasks to a group of kindergarten children. Tasks mastered by most children in kindergarten can then be designated as *kindergarten level skills*. By testing children at each grade level for which the inventory is designed, developmental information can be obtained that is useful in the interpretation of performance.

Educational Use of Locally Developed Assessment Instruments

Locally developed standardized tests can provide useful diagnostic information but generally do not provide sufficient information to identify the specific structural and functional aspects of a child's communication that cause it to be deficient. A locally developed communication skills inventory, however, can be used to compare a child's performance with that of peers in a variety of specific receptive and expressive communication skills. The information obtained from the inventory may be used to identify specific areas in which remediation is needed.

Locally developed assessment instruments are likely to meet the needs of bilingual students more adequately than any of the commercially available tests. No assessment instrument, however, is infallible. Therefore, speech–language pathologists and other members of the assessment team must be aware of the limitations of each assessment instrument so that the results are used appropriately in educational decision making.

Chapter 8

Educational Program Planning

Following the collection and analysis of the assessment data, the assessment team is faced with the complex task of determining how the child's needs can best be served. If it is determined that the child is an appropriate candidate for special education services (e.g., speech–language remediation), an individual education program must be developed for the student in which specific instructional goals and objectives are stated. In educational program planning for bilingual children with communicative disorders one must determine first, the child's specific educational needs; second, the appropriate special education programs that will meet those needs; and third, the appropriate language in which to teach the child.

What are the child's specific educational needs? A communicative disorder may occur in conjunction with a variety of other problems. The specific deficits that require special education intervention need to be delineated. The results of the speech–language evaluation should be reviewed in conjunction with assessment data obtained in other areas (e.g., academic achievement) so that a comprehensive educational program can be developed for the child. The most severe problems should receive the highest priority in educational program planning.

Deficits that can be attributed to the child's handicap must be distinguished from problems resulting from differences in the child's cultural and linguistic background. Special education intervention is appropriate only for those problems that result directly from the child's handicap. The educational placement that is most appropriate for the child should be based on the nature and severity of the handicapping conditions demonstrated by the child.

In what special education program(s) can the child's needs be met most effectively and efficiently? One hour of speech–language remediation weekly may be sufficient to meet the needs of some children, whereas others may require full-day placement in a special education classroom. Public Law 94-142 mandates that exceptional children be educated within the least restrictive environment. Thus, special education services are to be provided only to the extent to which a child's needs cannot be met within the regular classroom setting. Meyen (1978) described six specific elements that are central to the concept of education within the least restrictive environment.

> (1) assuming that a handicapped child can best be served through placement with nonhandicapped peers in regular class settings; (2) assigning primary instructional responsibility to regular class teachers; (3) providing support services to the regular class teacher as a means of helping the handicapped child when special assistance is required; (4) providing direct support services on a part-time basis to the handicapped child only if the regular class teacher is unable to provide an appropriate program through assistance from support personnel; (5) reserving assignment to special classes or separate programs as a last alternative; and (6) continually monitoring the child's progress, with the aim of returning the child to the regular class as soon as his or her performance suggests that such placement would be most appropriate. (p. 19)

The nature and severity of the problems demonstrated by the child should be considered in determining the type of special education program needed. Placement in a special education program is justified only when the resources in the regular education program are insufficient to meet the child's needs.

As mentioned previously, placement in remedial speech–language programs should be considered only when children demonstrate communicative behaviors that are atypical of other children who speak the same language and who have had similar cultural experiences. Limited English proficient children are not appropriate candidates for remedial speech–language programs if articulation and/or language problems are restricted to English—both languages must be affected.

In what language should instruction be provided? Because bilingual children with communicative disorders acquire language more slowly than their nonhandicapped peers, some special educators fear that these students may never learn English if instruction is provided in the minority language. Failure to acquire mastery of the first language, however, can impede both the child's cognitive and linguistic development.

> It has been found that the development of competence in the second language, that is, English, is partly a function of the type of competence already achieved in the first language at the time that instruction in the second begins. Children who do not master their first language will have difficulty developing skills in a second language and will also experience negative cognitive effects. (Juarez, 1983, p. 63)

It appears that instruction in the child's first language can promote the development of proficiency in both languages. Moreover, recent research has provided evidence that older children acquire a second language faster than younger children (Cummins, 1981; Krashen, Long & Scarcella, 1979; Skuttnabb-Kangas & Toukomaa, 1976).

We believe that remedial speech–language programs are most effective and efficient when limited English proficient children are provided with opportunities for instruction in their first language. Remediation provided in the handicapped child's first language can facilitate the development of proficiency in the second language. Rodrigo, a 5-year-old Spanish-speaking child who received speech–language remediation in a public school program, is described below to illustrate this phenomenon.

Rodrigo was identified as having a possible speech–language disorder during kindergarten screening. The classroom teacher reported that the child rarely spoke in the classroom and that his speech was quite difficult to understand. An interview with the parents revealed that Rodrigo used both English and Spanish when interacting with his 8-year-old brother. Both parents, however, used only Spanish in the home.

Testing was conducted in both English and Spanish. Although Rodrigo was able to name a variety of common nouns in both languages, he was not able to give the correct English label for the majority of the items that were correctly named in Spanish. This finding, in conjunction with data obtained from conversational communication samples and other measures, revealed that Spanish was Rodrigo's dominant language.

The results of testing in the dominant language indicated that Rodrigo's conversational communication consisted primarily of one- and two-word utterances. Moreover, the child's vocabulary was limited and multiple articulation errors were noted. When asked to repeat sentences after hearing them presented by the speech–language pathologist, Rodrigo consistently omitted a variety of grammatical constructions (e.g., plurals, articles, prepositions, verb forms). Examples of responses produced by the child are as follows:

Stimulus sentence	Rodrigo's response
El hombre está en la caja. (The man is in the box.)	Hombre caja. (Man box.)
Voy a la escuela. (I go to the school.)	Voy escuela. (I go school.)
Como en la casa. (I eat in the house).	Como casa. (I eat house).

The grammatical deficits observed during sentence imitation were typical of those produced by him during conversational speech. Thus, Rodrigo's mastery of the grammatical aspects of Spanish was quite limited.

Rodrigo was provided with three sessions of speech–language therapy weekly to improve vocabulary, sentence structure, speech sound production, and the functional use of language. All remedial instruction was provided in Spanish. During a 6-month period, progress was noted in all areas and the child began to use a variety of basic sentence types (e.g., present progressive) correctly in conversational speech.

Although Rodrigo's speech–language remediation program was provided entirely in Spanish, improved performance in English was also observed. Soon after Rodrigo started using the Spanish present progressive correctly when describing pictures (e.g., "El niño está comiendo"), correct productions of this construction in English were observed (e.g., "The boy is eating"). Similarly, improved articulation of speech sounds in Spanish (e.g., fricatives) was accompanied by improved production of similar sounds in English words.

The instructional activities provided in speech–language remediation programs may promote the development of language learning strategies that are common to all languages. Thus, by helping children to develop and use these strategies effectively in their dominant language, the task of learning a second language should be easier for them.

We have emphasized that remedial speech–language programs for limited English proficient children should provide instruction in the dominant language. We do not mean to imply, however, that it is never appropriate to incorporate both languages into a bilingual child's instructional program. Bilingual children with stuttering disorders, for example, often may require remediation in the minority language and in English if the problem is to be eliminated in both languages. It is recommended that remediation be provided in the child's dominant language first to provide the child with a sound basis in that language. In providing remediation for children with communicative disorders, Langdon (1983) made the following recommendation.

> When the teacher and other specialists feel the child has attained greater skills in Spanish or any native language, he or she could be slowly introduced to English. Having a sound basis in one language will enhance learning in the other. (p. 45)

In determining the extent to which the native language and English should be incorporated into the remedial program, assessment personnel must consider (1) the child's level of proficiency in the two languages, (2) the opportunities available for functional use of each language, and (3) the nature of the disorder requiring remediation. Also, one must not overlook the attitudes of the child's parents. Consultation with specialists in bilingual education is essential in determining how the minority language and English will be used in the child's instructional program.

Members of the assessment team must become familiar with the rationale for bilingual education and with the instructional techniques used in these programs if they are to use assessment data effectively in program planning for the bilingual child (Pacheco & Omark, 1984). Bilingual education programs provide an opportunity for limited English proficient children to receive instruction in their native language and to learn English as a second language.

The purpose of these programs is to maximize language minority children's opportunities for success within the educational system by providing a curriculum that is both culturally and linguistically appropriate.

Although the availability of bilingual education programs has grown rapidly in the United States, few of these programs are designed specifically for children with handicaps (Erickson & Walker, 1983; Grant, 1983). Mattes (1982c) found that few speech–language pathologists in Los Angeles County worked at schools where speech–language remediation was available to Spanish-dominant children in Spanish. Thus, there is a need for bilingual programs of instruction for handicapped, bilingual students in our schools.

PROGRAM PLACEMENT ALTERNATIVES

When a bilingual child is identified as having a communication disorder, the assessment team must determine the most beneficial educational placement for the child. A remedial program provided by a bilingual speech–language pathologist is the most desirable placement for children who require an intensive, individualized program of instruction. Other alternatives, however, need to be considered when the services of a bilingual speech–language pathologist cannot be obtained. The child's parents should always be provided with information about the program alternatives that are available.

Direct Services Provided by a Speech–Language Pathologist

Monolingual speech–language pathologists often provide remediation for bilingual, communicatively handicapped children who speak English as their dominant language. Problems often occur in planning and implementing instructional programs when the speech–language pathologist has no training in the area of bilingual language acquisition and/or is unfamiliar with the child's culture. Without this background, it is difficult to separate the abnormal aspects of the child's communication from those aspects that reflect cultural and/or linguistic differences. Moreover, speech–language pathologists who do not understand the child's culture may select instructional materials and teaching methods that are culturally inappropriate.

Speech–language pathologists from the dominant culture must become aware of and change their own ethnocentric stereotypes if they are to work effectively with individuals who have different cultural orientations. They also need to study the community, history, and way of life of the bilingual population being served (Pickering, 1976). In both program planning and implementation, monolingual speech–language pathologists should seek assistance from individuals who are familiar with the child's language and culture.

When remediation is necessary in a language other than English, the services of a bilingual speech–language pathologist should be obtained if at all possible. Bilingual speech–language pathologists who are from a cultural background different from that of bilingual children in the local community must have an understanding of the children's experiences, values, and learning styles so that culturally relevant instructional programs can be developed.

Local school systems should develop strategies for making the most effective use of any bilingual speech–language pathologists who are available. It may be possible, for example, to hire itinerant speech–language pathologists who are bilingual to provide remedial services for bilingual children in several school districts. It may also be possible for school districts to contract with bilingual speech–language pathologists in private practice who are able to come into the school specifically to work with bilingual children.

When a child's needs can be served most adequately in a setting outside of the school (e.g., community speech and hearing clinic), arrangements should be made, if possible, for remedial services within that setting. Contacts with local hospitals, private clinics, speech–language pathologists in private practice, university training programs, and other resources in the community may provide information that is helpful in locating a bilingual speech–language pathologist who can provide remedial services for bilingual students.

Consultation Model for Speech–Language Intervention

Frassinelli, Superior, and Meyers (1983) asserted that speech–language pathologists can meet the needs of more children by serving as consultants to classroom teachers. They defined consultation as "a three-person chain of services in which a consultant interacts with a caregiver (consultee) to benefit an individual (client) for whom the caregiver is responsible" (p. 25). In this approach the speech–language pathologist collaborates with the child's teacher in developing an individualized program of instruction for the child.

The needs of bilingual children with mild communicative disorders often can be met within the classroom if guidance in program planning is provided by the speech–language pathologist. The speech–language pathologist, for example, could suggest instructional activities for bilingual teachers and/or bilingual instructional aides to implement within the regular classroom. The speech–language pathologist may also have instructional materials (e.g., stimulus pictures) that could be used to provide classroom instructional activities.

Parents can also participate in program implementation by providing instruction in the home under the guidance of the speech–language pathologist. By consulting with both the classroom teacher and the child's parents, remediation can be provided in contexts where the child has frequent opportunities for the functional use of language. Lombardino and Mangan (1983) found that parents who had been trained to provide language instruction were effective in improving the language skills of their children.

The consultation model for speech–language intervention is often the most appropriate approach when children demonstrate mild communicative disorders that do not require an intensive remedial program. Bilingual classroom teachers, however, cannot be expected to meet the needs of all limited English proficient children in their classrooms who demonstrate communicative disorders. Other alternatives are needed for children who require more attention than that which can be expected within the regular education curriculum.

Paraprofessionals and Program Implementation

The use of trained bilingual paraprofessionals to implement remedial speech–language programs should be considered when the supply of bilingual speech–language pathologists is insufficient to meet the local demand. Bilingual paraprofessionals hired specifically to work in speech–language programs can be trained to provide remediation for a variety of types of communicative disorders.

Programs administered by paraprofessionals should be structured so that they specify precisely the behavior required of both the paraprofessional and the child. Thus, the paraprofessional's task is to present instructions, stimulus materials, social reinforcement, and so forth, in the manner specified within the program.

Paraprofessionals have proven to be effective in providing remediation when programmed instruction is used (Costello & Schoen, 1978; Harris, 1975). Paraprofessionals, for example, can be trained to administer structured articulation programs in which the child must reach a predetermined performance criteria at each program step before progressing to the next step of the program. Skill in using programmed materials can be acquired quickly by paraprofessionals.

> Paraprofessionals can be trained to administer programmed instruction in a matter of hours. Critical lesson-planning decisions are made by the professional speech and language clinician when the program is designed or when a commercially available program is selected. The paraprofessional then needs only to learn relatively simple concepts beyond following the program's format, such as recognizing correct and incorrect responses, presenting the proper consequences for correct and incorrect responses, and recording responses as correct or incorrect. (Costello & Schoen, 1978, p. 119)

The limited training of paraprofessionals must be recognized when they are used to administer remedial programs. A paraprofessional who has been trained only to work with children who demonstrate mild articulation disorders, for example, is not qualified to provide remediation for an autistic child with minimal language capabilities and a severe behavior disorder. Paraprofessionals should be used only when the speech–language pathologist is certain that they have the training necessary to provide instruction that will be effective in meeting children's needs.

The primary responsibility of the paraprofessional in the remediation process is that of *implementing* instructional programs. They should never be assigned the responsibility for planning instructional programs or writing educational objectives. The speech–language pathologist must be involved in program planning. Specialists in bilingual education, classroom teachers, and bilingual assessment personnel are among those who can assist monolingual speech–language pathologists both in developing instructional programs that can be implemented by bilingual paraprofessionals and in evaluating the effectiveness of those programs.

ASSESSMENT AS AN ONGOING PROCESS

Cooperation among members of the assessment team is vital throughout both program planning and implementation. Assessment must be an ongoing process if instructional programs are to be effective in meeting children's changing needs. An ongoing approach to assessment makes it possible to monitor student progress at regular intervals and to modify the instructional program when changes are needed.

Lerner (1976) asserted that "team approaches are often interdisciplinary in name only; certain team members or disciplines are not accorded equal status in diagnosis, and the teamwork is not carried through in therapy" (p. 363). The development of effective remedial programs for bilingual, bicultural children with communicative disorders requires the combined efforts of individuals from both bilingual education and special education.

By developing and implementing an interdisciplinary team approach to assessing and remediating communicative disorders in bilingual student populations, programs can be provided that are both culturally and linguistically relevant. Members of the team must strive to increase instructional options so that the diverse needs of handicapped bilingual children can be met. A variety of instructional options should be considered when planning educational programs for individual children.

Consideration of individual differences is necessary in both assessment and program planning. Bilingual children cannot all be evaluated using the same tests and their problems cannot all be treated in the same way. While some children with communicative disorders may be served adequately when their regular classroom program is modified, others need to be served in remedial speech–language programs and/or in other special education placements. By individualizing approaches to assessment and by using the assessment data in a nondiscriminatory manner, instructional programs can be developed that are effective in helping bilingual children with communicative disorders to conquer their handicaps and reach their full potential.

Appendix A

Guidelines for Interviewing Parents About Cultural and Environmental Influences

After talking with community members about the general cultural characteristics of the community, it is still necessary to discover what experiences each child has had. The following set of questions can be used to find out about the direct cultural and environmental experiences of the child so that appropriate educational programs can be planned.

1. What language(s) do the parents speak to each other?
2. What language(s) do the parents speak to the child?
3. What language(s) do the children use with each other?
4. What language does the referred child prefer to use when playing with friends?
5. Who takes care of the child after school? What language is used?
6. Who lives in the home (parents, grandparents, etc.)?
7. How much time does each parent have to interact with the child?
8. With whom does the child play when at home?
9. What television programs are seen in each language?
10. Are stories read to the child? In what language is the reading material written?
11. What language is used in church services, if attended?
12. What does the child do after school and on weekends?
13. What responsibilities does the child have in the home?
14. How is the child expected to act toward parents, teachers, and other adults?
15. In what cultural activities does the family participate?
16. How do the parents expect adults to act toward the child?

17. Are there any specific prohibitions in the everyday interactions between adults and children, for example, do not look adults in the eye when talking to them, do not pat children on the top of the head, do not ask children questions?
18. How long has the family been in this country?
19. How long has the family been in the local community?
20. How much contact does the family have with the homeland? What kind of contact?

Appendix B

Test Descriptions and Publishers' Addresses

Descriptive information about many of the speech and language assessment instruments available for speakers of Spanish and other minority languages has been published (see Cole & Campbell-Calloway, 1983; Cole & Snope, 1981; Day et al., 1981; McCollum & Day, 1981; Watson, Grouell, Heller, & Omark, 1981). This appendix is limited to a selected sample of instruments currently being used in the assessment of Spanish-speaking children.

REVIEW OF FOUR NEW ASSESSMENT INSTRUMENTS

Detailed reviews of four recently published assessment instruments are presented in this section to illustrate both norm-referenced and criterion-referenced approaches to assessment. All four of the measures were published between 1980 and 1984.

Norm-Referenced Testing

Title of instrument:	Prueba del Desarrollo Inicial del Lenguaje
Developed by:	Wayne P. Hresko, D. Kim Reid, and Donald D. Hammill
Available from:	Pro-Ed 5341 Industrial Oaks Blvd. Austin, TX 78735
Age range:	Ages 3–0 to 7–11
Description:	

The Prueba del Desarrollo Inicial del Lenguaje is a 38-item test of receptive and expressive language skills. The test assesses both form (the structural aspects of language) and content (the ability to encode and decode meaning). Tasks requiring the child to answer questions about pictures, repeat sentences, describe noun functions, define words, and point to pictures named by the examiner are among the measures included on the test. The instrument can be used to identify children in need of more extensive clinical appraisal for possible communicative disorders.

The Prueba del Desarrollo Inicial del Lenguaje follows a format similar to that used on the Test of Early Language Development (Hresko, Reid, & Hammill, 1981), a test for English-speaking children. Some of the items are direct translations of items on the Test of Early Language Development, whereas others differ in content.

The test was standardized on a sample of 549 Spanish-speaking children. Countries represented in the sample were Mexico (127 children), Puerto Rico (250 children), and the United States (172 children). The specific criteria used in selecting subjects for the standardization sample are not described in the test manual.

Scores on the test are reported as language quotients and percentiles. Separate norm tables are provided for Mexico, Puerto Rico, and the United States. Combined norms for the entire subject sample are also presented.

The test's internal consistency reliability was found to be within acceptable limits (above .85) at all age levels; no other reliability data are reported.

A study of 20 children with identified language deficiencies revealed that scores on the test can be used to distinguish between groups of children with language problems and those known to be without such difficulties. The extent to which performance on this measure correlates with performance on other measures of Spanish language proficiency is not reported.

Because limited information is provided about the test standardization population, potential users of the test have no way of determining the appropriateness of the normative data for individual children who are administered the instrument. Moreover, the standardization sample in each of the three countries was small. A review of the child's performance on individual test items can provide indications of possible problems that are being experienced by the child in understanding and/or using the language. Further information on the validity of the instrument is needed.

Title of instrument:	Pruebas de Expresión Oral y Percepción de la Lengua Española
Developed by:	Sharen Mares, Project Manager
Available from:	Division of Support Services Office of the Los Angeles County Superintendent of Public Schools 9300 East Imperial Highway Downey, CA 90242
Age range:	Age 6–0 through 9–11

Description:

Pruebas de Expresión Oral y Percepción de la Lengua Española is an example of a language measure developed within the public schools for use in assessing a specific population of Spanish-speaking children. This instrument is appropriate only for predominantly Spanish-speaking children of Mexican descent living in Southern California. The five subtests included in this measure are (1) Auditory Sequential Memory, (2) Auditory Association, (3) Encoding, (4) Story Comprehension, and (5) Sentence Repetition. The entire test is administered in Spanish.

The test was developed "for the purpose of assessing language abilities and disabilities of Mexican and Mexican American children living in Southern California" (p. 3). The instrument was standardized in Southern California on a stratified sample of 674 predominantly Spanish-speaking students from Los Angeles, Santa Barbara, Orange, San Diego, and Imperial Counties. All students in the sample were judged by their teachers as demonstrating average or above average performance in classroom oral language activities. Moreover, none of the children were receiving speech–language remediation or other special education services.

The child's raw score for each subtest is converted to a scale score. Percentiles are not currently available but will become available in the future.

All five subtests were found to fall within acceptable limits of reliability. The reliability measures studied were internal consistency, test–retest reliability, interscorer reliability, and vertical equating of item difficulty.

The validity of the test was determined primarily through the inspection of test content by "recognized authorities" (p. 11). The test manual includes detailed tables showing data obtained from factor analysis, subtest intercorrelations, and subtest-to-total-test intercorrelations. The validity of the test for use in distinguishing normal from communicatively handicapped children is not reported in the test manual. The instrument is still in an experimental version and, therefore, caution must be exercised in the use of the test results.

Title of instrument:	Woodcock Spanish Psycho-Educational Battery
Developed by:	Richard W. Woodcock
Available from:	Teaching Resources 50 Pond Park Road Hingham, MA 02043
Age range:	Age 3 through adult

Description:

The Woodcock Spanish Psycho-Educational Battery is designed for use in assessing the cognitive ability and scholastic achievement of Spanish-speaking individuals. The test can be used to measure discrepancies between potential and achievement and to identify individuals with specific learning deficits.

The instrument includes 17 subtests:

1. Picture Vocabulary
2. Spatial Relations
3. Visual Auditory Learning
4. Quantitative Concepts
5. Visual Matching
6. Antonyms–Synonyms
7. Analysis–Synthesis
8. Numbers Reversed
9. Concept Formation
10. Analogies
11. Letter Word Identification
12. Word Attack
13. Passage Comprehension
14. Calculation
15. Applied Problems
16. Dictation
17. Proofing

These 17 subtests are among the 24 subtests included in the Woodcock–Johnson Psycho-Educational Battery (Woodcock & Johnson, 1977), a test designed for English speakers. To avoid the problems inherent in direct translation, modifications were made in the content of language items on the Spanish version of the test.

The eight subtests measuring oral language, reading, and written language can be obtained separately in the Woodcock Language Proficiency Battery—Spanish form (Woodcock, 1982). This battery includes the following subtests:

1. Picture Vocabulary
2. Antonyms–Synonyms
3. Analogies
4. Letter–Word Identification
5. Word Attack
6. Passage Comprehension
7. Dictation
8. Proofing

The results of the Woodcock Spanish Psycho-Educational Battery are interpreted based on clusters of subtests. The Oral Language Cluster is of special interest in the assessment of individuals with possible communicative disorders. Subtests included in this cluster are Picture Vocabulary, Antonyms–Synonyms, and Analogies.

A full variety of scores (e.g., percentile ranks, grade equivalents, age equivalents, standard scores) are provided to facilitate interpretation of test results. The Response Booklet includes a Percentile Rank Profile, Subtest Profile, Achievement–Aptitude Profile, and an Instructional Implications Profile.

The Woodcock Spanish Psycho-Educational Battery provides General Spanish Norms that were obtained on a sample of 802 children representing Costa Rica, Mexico, Peru, Puerto Rico, and Spain. Equated U.S. Norms are in preparation and will make it possible to compare the Spanish speaker's performance with that of English speakers in the United States.

It is not felt that the General Spanish Norms or the Equated U.S. Norms provide sufficient information for the identification of individuals with specific learning deficits. The standardization sample for the General Spanish Norms was quite heterogeneous. Norms are needed so that student performance can be compared to that of others who have had similar cultural and linguistic experiences.

The technical manual for the Woodcock Spanish Psycho-Educational Battery has not yet been released. Thus, reliability and validity data are not available at this time.

The information obtained from the Woodcock Spanish Psycho-Educational Battery should be useful in identifying specific strengths and weaknesses in the performance of Spanish-speaking students. The subtests in the Oral Language Cluster of the battery, however, are limited to the assessment of cognitive–semantic processing and require only one-word responses from the student. Thus, these subtests sample only a small aspect of the individual's oral language capabilities.

Criterion-Referenced Testing

Title of instrument:	BRIGANCE® Assessment of Basic Skills—Spanish Edition
Developed by:	Albert H. Brigance
Available from:	Curriculum Associates, Inc. 5 Esquire Road North Billerica, MA 01862-2589
Age range:	Prekindergarten through Grade 8

Description:

The Assessment of Basic Skills includes 102 criterion-referenced tests in the areas of (1) Readiness, (2) Speech, (3) Functional Word Recognition, (4) Oral Reading, (5) Reading Comprehension, (6) Word Analysis, (7) Listening, (8) Writing and Alphabetizing, (9) Numbers and Computation, and (10) Measurement. The instrument is an adaptation of the Comprehensive Inventory of Basic Skills (Brigance, 1983), an inventory designed for English-speaking children.

The Assessment of Basic Skills offers an efficient system for recording the results of the testing and tracking student progress. Forms for record keeping include the Student Record Book, Class Record Book, Kindergarten through Sixth-Grade Screening Forms, and the Dominant Language Screening Form.

The author states that "the assessment procedures are simple; many can be given, with supervision, by an aide adept in the Spanish language" (p. vi). Guidelines are not provided, however, for the selection or use of aides in test administration.

The inventory was reviewed for content validity by authorities in Spanish translation, linguists, and educators. The content validity was also evaluated by over 150 professionals who field-tested the instrument. Bilingual special education teachers, speech–language pathologists, and bilingual education teachers were among those who participated in the field testing. Changes were made in the inventory based on the information obtained. Content validity is the only validity measure reported. Moreover, data on the reliability of the individual criterion-referenced tests are not provided.

The assessments in the Speech section of the inventory are designed to provide teachers and others with information for use in (1) identifying children who should be referred for special testing, (2) determining instructional objectives, and (3) tracking student progress. The author specifically states that "the assessments have not been designed to provide precise quantitative measures that can be used to make a clinical diagnosis of specific speech problems" (p. 39).

The Readiness, Speech, and Listening sections of the Assessment of Basic Skills each contain tasks that can be used in the speech–language assessment of Spanish-speaking children. Directional and positional concepts, colors, body parts, articulation of initial and final sounds, sentence memory, listening comprehension, and sentence structure are among the skills assessed.

A picture-naming task is used to assess production of speech sounds in the initial and final position of words. Phonemes that are represented by more than one letter in printed Spanish words are assessed as if they were distinct sounds. Thus, although the letters *s* and *z* represent the same sound, the inventory includes items specifically designed to assess articulation of *s* and items specifically designed to assess articulation of *z*.

The Dominant Language Screening Form is used when information about the child's relative proficiency in English and Spanish is needed. The results of selected listening, speaking, and reading measures that can be administered in both English and Spanish are recorded on this form. One of the 10 criterion-referenced measures used in the language dominance screening is Sentence Memory. This task requires the child to repeat sentences after hearing them read by the examiner. Sentence length is based on the number of syllables rather than the number of words in the sentence. Although matched for syllable length, the English sentences contain more words than the Spanish sentences. The shortest of the two 10-syllable English sentences, for example, is nine words in length while the shortest 10-syllable Spanish sentence is only four words in length. Thus, it seems unlikely that these two tasks are equivalent in difficulty. When examining language dominance, the information recorded on the Dominant Language Screening Form should be used in conjunction with other data.

Although the information obtained from the inventory is not precise enough for the clinical diagnosis of specific communicative disorders, the results can be helpful to speech–language pathologists and other school personnel in program planning. The Assessment of Basic Skills is a comprehensive, well-organized inventory that can provide useful information about Spanish-speaking children's performance in a variety of areas. Further research, however, is needed to assess the reliability and validity of the individual criterion-referenced tests.

Appropriateness of the Assessment Instruments

The norm-referenced tests described previously illustrate several different procedures that have been used in standardizing measures for use in the assessment of Spanish-speaking children. The Prueba del Desarrollo Inicial del Lenguaje (Hresko et al., 1982) includes separate norms for three different countries while the Woodcock Spanish Psycho-Educational Battery (Woodcock, 1982) combines normative data obtained from five different countries. In contrast, Pruebas de Expresión Oral y Percepción de la Lengua Española (Mares, 1980) includes norms only for Spanish-speaking children in Southern California.

Because of the heterogeneity of the Spanish-speaking population, care must be taken in the selection of an appropriate test instrument whenever tests are used. Test norms obtained outside of the United States can lead to misdiagnosis if used to interpret the performance of Spanish-speaking children who were born in this country. Moreover, norms obtained within the United States must always be examined to determine their appropriateness for use in interpreting test data obtained when children from the local population are assessed.

The Assessment of Basic Skills (Brigance, 1984) is an example of an instrument that can serve as an alternative to norm-referenced tests. This criterion-referenced inventory can be used to measure the extent to which the child has mastered specific speech and language skills. Without developmental information on the speech and language skills tested, however, assessment personnel may experience difficulty in interpreting test performance.

Both norm-referenced and criterion-referenced assessment instruments should always be field-tested on students from the local population prior to use in the assessment of children with suspected communication disorders. Moreover, assessment instruments should be judged in terms of their appropriateness for each child who is assessed.

BRIEF DESCRIPTIONS OF 14 ASSESSMENT INSTRUMENTS

It is beyond the scope of this book to provide detailed descriptions of all speech and language assessment instruments currently available for use in assessing Spanish-speaking individuals. Brief descriptions of 14 of these instruments follow.

Title of instrument:	Austin Spanish Articulation Test
Developed by:	Elizabeth Carrow

Available from: Teaching Resources
50 Pond Park Road
Hingham, MA 02043

Age range: Ages 4 and up.

Description:

The Austin Spanish Articulation Test is designed for use in assessing children's productions of consonants, vowels, diphthongs, and clusters in isolated words. For each sound tested, the individual is presented with a picture and read a sentence in which the final word is missing. The child's task is to complete the sentence. The Austin Spanish Articulation Test was field-tested on 29 children in Texas. Norms are not provided.

Title of instrument: Ber-Sil Spanish Test

Developed by: Marjorie L. Beringer

Available from: The Ber-Sil Company
3412 Seaglen Drive
Rancho Palos Verdes, CA 90274

Age range: Ages 4 through 12

Description:

The Ber-Sil Spanish Test is designed for use as a screening measure. The test assesses the child's understanding of 100 Spanish vocabulary words, responses to 13 simple verbal directions, and visual motor ability (drawing and writing). Norms, obtained in Los Angeles County, are provided only for the vocabulary comprehension portion of the test. All verbal stimuli for the test are presented on tape. Therefore, it is not necessary to speak Spanish to administer the test.

Title of instrument: Bilingual Syntax Measure

Developed by: Marine Burt, Heidi Dulay, and Eduardo Hernandez-Chavez

Available from: The Psychological Corporation
757 Third Ave.
New York, NY 10017

Age range: Level 1: Grades K–2
Level 2: Grades 3 and up

Description:

The Bilingual Syntax Measure is designed to measure syntactic production in both English and Spanish and can be used as a language dominance test.

The child is placed at one of five levels of proficiency in each language based on the score obtained. Norms are not provided.

Title of instrument: Boehm Test of Basic Concepts

Developed by: Ann E. Boehm

Available from: The Psychological Corporation
757 Third Ave.
New York, NY 10017

Age range: Grades K–2

Description:

The Boehm Test of Basic Concepts is a screening measure of the child's comprehension of 50 basic concepts. The Spanish version of the test is a literal translation of the English version. Norms are not available for the Spanish translation.

Title of instrument: Del Rio Language Screening Test

Developed by: Allen S. Toronto, D. Leverman, Cornelia Hanna, Peggy Rosenzweig, and Antoneta Maldonado

Available from: National Educational Laboratory Publishers, Inc.
PO Box 1003
Austin, TX 78767

Age range: Ages 3–0 through 6–11

Description:

The Del Rio Language Screening Test includes screening measures in both English and Spanish to assess receptive vocabulary, sentence repetition (length), sentence repetition (complexity), memory for oral commands, and story comprehension. Norms were obtained in Del Rio, Texas, for three separate groups: (1) English-speaking Anglo Americans, (2) predominantly English-speaking Mexican Americans, and (3) predominantly Spanish-speaking Mexican Americans.

Title of instrument: Dos Amigos Verbal Language Scales

Developed by: Donald E. Critchlow

Available from: Academic Therapy Publications
1539 Fourth St.
PO Box 899
San Rafael, CA 94901

Age range:	Grades K–6
Description:	

The Dos Amigos Verbal Language Scales are designed for use as a language dominance measure. The child's task is to give verbal opposites for English and Spanish words presented by the examiner. The test was normed on Mexican American children in Southern Texas.

Title of instrument:	Examines para Diagnosticar Impedimentos de Afasia
Developed by:	Lilian Rojas Moncada and Mary Marshall
Available from:	Pinnacle Press PO Box 1122 Murfreesboro, TN 37130
Age range:	Primarily for adolescents and adults
Description:	

This instrument is a Spanish adaptation of the Aphasia Language Performance Scales. Scales measuring listening, speaking, reading, and writing are included in the test. The severity of the aphasic client's impairment is determined separately for each scale. Norms are not provided.

Title of instrument:	Language Assessment Scales, Level 1
Developed by:	Edward A. DeAvila and Sharon E. Duncan
Available from:	Linguametrics Group PO Box 454 Corte Madera, CA 94925
Age range:	Grades K–5
Description:	

The Language Assessment Scales are designed to assess auditory discrimination, vocabulary, phoneme production, sentence comprehension, and oral production (storytelling) in both English and Spanish. The total score is used to place the child at one of five levels of proficiency in each language tested. The child's dominant language is determined based on a comparison of performance in English and Spanish. The Spanish portion of the Language Assessment Scales was normed on children from Mexican American, Latin American, and Puerto Rican backgrounds. The English portion was normed on English-speaking children in the Southwest.

Title of instrument: Medida Española de Articulación (La "Meda")

Developed by: Marilyn Aldrich Mason, Blanche Figueroa Smith, and Mary Martinez Henshaw

Available from: San Ysidro School District
4350 Otay Mesa Road
San Ysidro, CA 92073

Age range: Ages 4–0 to 9–0

Description:

This instrument is designed for use in assessing articulation of single words in Spanish. Pictures and stimulus sentences read by the examiner are used to elicit the child's responses. Normative data were obtained on Mexican American children in San Ysidro, California.

Title of instrument: Screening Test of Spanish Grammar

Developed by: Allen S. Toronto

Available from: Northwestern University Press
1735 Benson Ave.
Evanston, IL 60201

Age range: Ages 3–0 to 6–11

Description:

The Screening Test of Spanish Grammar is designed for use in screening Spanish-speaking children for possible syntactic deficits in Spanish. The instrument consists of two subtests, one testing comprehension and one testing production. The two subtests each assess 23 identical syntactic structures. The test was normed on children of Mexican and Puerto Rican descent living in Chicago, Illinois.

Title of instrument: Southwestern Spanish Articulation Test

Developed by: Allen S. Toronto

Available from: National Educational Laboratory Publishers, Inc.
PO Box 1003
Austin, TX 78757

Age range: Age 3 and up

Description:

The Southwestern Spanish Articulation Test uses a picture-naming task to assess articulation of words in isolation. All Spanish consonants are assessed in initial. medial, and final word position. Norms are not provided.

Title of instrument: Spanish Language Assessment Procedures: A Communication Skills Inventory

Developed by: Larry J. Mattes

Available from: Academic Communication Associates
PO Box 6044
Oceanside, CA 92056

Age range: Grades K–3

Description:

This inventory is designed for use in assessing both the structural and functional aspects of communication. Articulation, language, voice, and fluency are examined. Criterion-referenced tasks and naturalistic observation techniques are used to collect the assessment data. Record forms for recording students' performance and tracking their progress are included. When used within the regular classroom setting, a child's performance can be compared to the local peer group. Norms for the articulation measure were obtained on Mexican American children in Southern California. No other normative information is presented.

Title of instrument: Test for Auditory Comprehension of Language

Developed by: Elizabeth Carrow

Available from: Teaching Resources
50 Pond Park Road
Hingham, MA 02043

Age range: Ages 3–0 to 6–11

Description:

The Test for Auditory Comprehension of Language assesses comprehension of form classes and function words, morphological constructions, grammatical categories, and syntactic structures in English and Spanish. The Spanish version is a direct translation of the English version and is not normed. Norms are provided for the English version of the instrument.

Title of instrument: Toronto Tests of Receptive Vocabulary

Developed by: Allen S. Toronto

Available from: National Educational Laboratory Publishers, Inc.
PO Box 1003
Austin, TX 78767

Age range: Ages 4–0 to 10–11

Description:

The Toronto Tests of Receptive Vocabulary are designed for use in assessing receptive vocabulary proficiency in English and Spanish. The results can be used to identify Spanish- and English-speaking children whose understanding of vocabulary is significantly below that of their peer group. Separate norms are provided for Anglo American children, English-speaking Mexican American children, and Spanish-speaking Mexican American children. These norms were obtained in San Antonio, San Marcos, and Temple, Texas.

Appendix C

Test Evaluation Form*

Title of Test:

Author:

Publisher:

Date of Publication:

DIRECTIONS FOR COMPLETING THIS FORM: Evaluate the test in each of the areas below using the following scoring system:

G = Good F = Fair P = Poor
NI = No Information NA = Not Applicable

I. PURPOSES OF THE TEST

______ A. The purposes of the test are described adequately in the test manual.

______ B. The purposes of the test are appropriate for the intended local uses of the instrument.

Comments:

II. CONSTRUCTION OF THE TEST

______ A. Test was developed based on a contemporary theoretical model of speech–language development and reflects the findings of recent research.

*This form may be reproduced for local use.

_____ B. Procedures used in developing test content (e.g., selection and field-testing of test items) were adequate.

Comments:

III. PROCEDURES

A. Procedures for test administration:

_____ 1. Described adequately in the test manual.

_____ 2. Appropriate for the local population.

B. Procedures for scoring the test:

_____ 1. Described adequately in the test manual.

_____ 2. Appropriate for the local population.

C. Procedures for test interpretation:

_____ 1. Described adequately in the test manual.

_____ 2. Appropriate for the local population.

Comments:

IV. LINGUISTIC APPROPRIATENESS OF THE TEST

_____ A. Directions presented to the child are written in the dialect used by the local population.

_____ B. Test items are written in the dialect used by the local population.

Comments:

V. CULTURAL APPROPRIATENESS OF THE TEST

_____ A. Types of tasks that the child is asked to perform are culturally appropriate for the local population.

_____ B. Content of test items is culturally appropriate for the local population.

______ C. Visual stimuli (e.g., stimulus pictures used on the test) are culturally appropriate for the local population.

Comments:

VI. ADEQUACY OF NORMS

______ A. Procedures for selection of the standardization sample are described in detail.

______ B. Standardization sample is an appropriate comparison group for the local population in terms of:

______ 1. Age
______ 2. Ethnic background
______ 3. Place of birth
______ 4. Community of current residence
______ 5. Length of residency in the United States
______ 6. Socioeconomic level
______ 7. Language classification (e.g., limited English proficient)
______ 8. Language most often used by child at home.
______ 9. Language most often used by child at school.
______ 10. Type of language program provided in school setting (e.g., bilingual education)

Comments:

VII. ADEQUACY OF TEST RELIABILITY DATA

______ A. Test–retest reliability
______ B. Alternate form rcliability
______ C. Split-half or internal consistency

Comments:

VIII. ADEQUACY OF TEST VALIDITY DATA

______ A. Face validity

______ B. Content validity

______ C. Construct validity

______ D. Concurrent validity

______ E. Predictive validity

Comments:

Appendix D

Characteristics of Minority Languages Spoken in the United States

This appendix presents structural descriptions of 15 minority languages. The language descriptions, from Ruhlen (1976),* can serve as a starting point for discussions between speech–language pathologists, bilingual education teachers, paraprofessionals, and others. The languages represented are those most frequently used by limited English proficient children in the United States (see Erickson & Walker, 1983). The information presented in the descriptions should be useful to speech–language pathologists in their efforts to distinguish differences from disorders. The information should also be of value when tests need to be constructed in the child's native language.

PHONETIC SYMBOLS IN THE LANGUAGE DESCRIPTIONS

The 4 phonetic transcription charts that appear on the following pages illustrate each of the symbols used to represent speech sounds in the language descriptions. The charts present (1) symbols for the consonants, (2) symbols for the vowels, (3) symbols for the glides, and (4) diacritical markings.

1. *Consonants.* The *consonant chart* summarizes the most essential characteristics of the consonants. The consonants are organized in columns according to *place of articulation* (bilabial, labiodental, interdental, etc.) and in rows according to *acoustical classification* (stops, affricates, fricatives, etc.). Voiceless consonants always appear directly above their voiced counterparts. The voiceless bilabial stop *p*, for example, is presented directly above its voiced counterpart, *b*.

2. *Vowels.* The *vowel diagram* illustrates the tongue and lip position for each vowel. The terms *high, lower-high, mid, lower-mid,* and *low* refer to the extent of tongue

*The language descriptions and phonetic transcription charts in this appendix are reprinted with permission from M. Ruhlen, *Guide to the languages of the world.* An additional 700 languages appear in the *Guide,* available from Los Amigos Research Associates, 7035 Galewood, San Diego, CA 92120 ($15.00 per copy).

elevation while the terms *front, central,* and *back* refer to the portion of the tongue that is critically involved in producing the sound. The degree of lip rounding for each vowel is also illustrated in the diagram.

3. *Glides.* Descriptions of the glides in terms of tongue elevation (*high* or *mid*), location (*front, central* or *back*), and lip rounding (*rounded* or *unrounded*) are presented below the *vowel diagram.*

4. *Diacritics.* This chart is a list of diacritical markings. The use of diacritical markings makes it possible to indicate how the production of individual phonemes varies in different languages. The phoneme *p*, for example, is generally aspirated in English. Therefore, the phoneme appears as p^h in the language description for English to indicate that it is generally aspirated. The symbols used in the language descriptions represent the phonemes as they most often are produced within the language; other variations in the production of particular phonemes (i.e., allophones) may occur.

PHONETIC TRANSCRIPTION

The following is a list of phonetic symbols for all the speech sounds cited in Part II:

1 CONSONANTS

	Bilabial	Labiodental	Interdental	Dental	Alveolar	Retroflex	Palatal*	Velar	Labial-Velar	Uvular	Pharyngeal	Glottal
Stops	p b			t̪ d̪	t d	ṭ ḍ	c ɟ	k g	k͡p g͡b	q ɢ		ʔ
Affricates	pᶠ	t̪θ d̪ð	t̪s d̪z	ts tˡ dz dˡ	č̣ ǰ̣	č cç ǰ ɟʝ̂	kx gˡ				
Fricatives	ɸ β	f v	θ ð	s̪ z̪	s z	ṣ ʃ̣ ẓ ʒ̣	ʃ ç ʒ ʝ̂	x ɣ		χ ʁ	ħ ʕ	h ɦ
Approximants		ʋ		ɹ̪	ɹ	ɹ̣	j		w			
Nasals	m			n̪	n	ṇ	ɲ	ŋ	m͡ŋ	ɴ		
Laterals				l̪	l ɬ	ḷ	ʎ					
Trills				r̪	r	ṛ				ʀ		
Flaps				ɾ̪	ɾ	ɾ̣						
Ejectives	pʔ			t̪ʔ	tʔ		cʔ	kʔ	k͡pʔ	qʔ		
Implosives	ɓ ʔb			ɗ̪ ʔd	ɗ ʔd		ʄ ʔɟ	ɠ ʔg				
Clicks	q			ł ǂ	ʒ	C						

*Includes both palatal and palato-alveolar sounds.

2 VOWELS

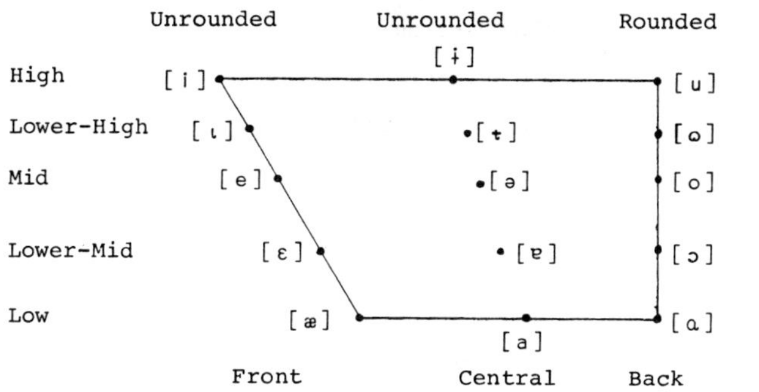

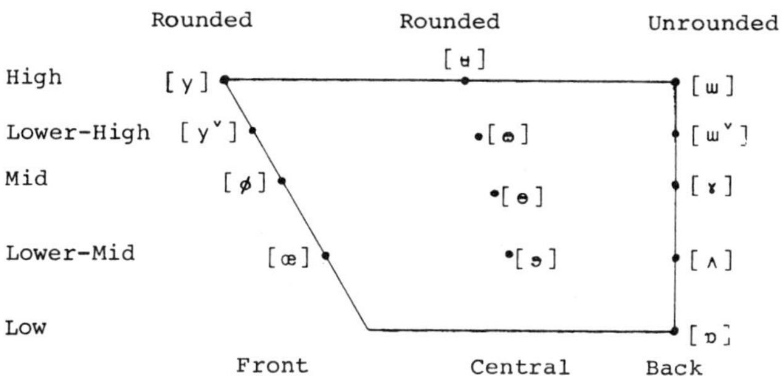

3 GLIDES

[j]: High front unrounded
[ɥ]: High front rounded
[w]: High back rounded
[ɯ̯]: High back unrounded
[e̯]: Mid front unrounded
[ə̯]: Mid central unrounded
[o̯]: Mid back rounded

4 DIACRITICS

[ʰ]: Aspirated
[˜]: Nasalized
[¯]: Long
[̪]: Dental
[̣]: Retroflex
[̱]: Fortis
[̥]: Voiceless
[̤]: Breathy Voice
[̰]: Creaky Voice
[ˀ]: Ejective/Preglottalized

N: Nasal (m, n, ŋ)
L: Liquid (l, r, ɹ)
G: Glide (j, w)
N: North
E: East
S: South
W: West
C: Central

[ᶢ]: Voiced Click

[⁀]: Coarticulated

[̩]: Syllabic

[ʲ]: Palatalized

[ʷ]: Labialized

[ᵚ]: Velarized

[ˁ]: Pharyngealized

[ɬ]: Voiceless Lateral Fricative

[ɮ]: Voiced Lateral Fricative

[ľ]: Lateral Flap

[ ]: Phonetic Transcription

/ /: Phonemic Transcription

CONTENT OF THE LANGUAGE DESCRIPTIONS

General information about the language

Each of the language descriptions begins with general information about the language as shown below for English:

ENGLISH (American) [Gleason 1961] [Indo-European: Germanic: West] [United States; 300 million]

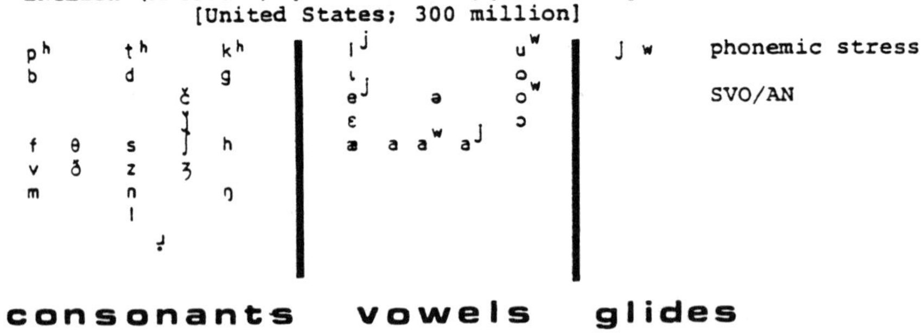

The general information categories included in the language descriptions are as follows.

Category	Example for English
Name of the language	English
Name of the dialect	American
Source of the phonetic information*	Gleason 1961
Language classification	Indo-European: Germanic: West

*These references appear in Ruhlen (1976).

Primary country where language is used	United States
Approximate number of speakers of the language worldwide	300 million

Phonemes

The consonants, vowels, and glides are presented for each language. The arrangement of the consonants closely parallels their position on the *consonant chart* described earlier. Likewise, the vowels are arranged to reflect their position on the *vowel diagram*. The language descriptions should be used in conjunction with the *consonant chart* and with the *vowel diagram* when information is needed about the characteristics of individual phonemes.

Tones

The oriental languages (Cantonese, Japanese, Korean, Mandarin, Vietnamese) are *tone* languages. The tones influence the acoustical characteristics of vowels. The characteristics of these tones (e.g., high rising, low dropping) are presented for the tone languages.

Syllable Types

The sequences in which consonants and vowels can be arranged within syllables are presented only for languages that use a restricted variety of syllable types. Most of the European languages have so many possibilities that no syllable order is listed.

The symbols used in the language descriptions to illustrate the syllable types are as follows:

C = consonant that is mandatory;
(C) = consonant that may occur but does not always occur in a particular context;
V = vowel that is mandatory.

These symbols are arranged in the order in which they occur within syllables. Tagalog, for example, uses the following syllable type: (C) CV (C). Thus, Tagalog has a basic CV (consonant followed by vowel) syllable which sometimes is preceded by and/or followed by a consonant.

Stress Patterns

Some languages tend to emphasize particular stress patterns within words. The specific stress pattern that is used in the language (e.g., nonphonemic stress) is stated in the language description.

Word Order

The order of the subject (S), verb (V), and object (O) in simple sentences is presented for each language. In English, for example, the basic word order is as follows: The boy (S) eats (V) cake (O). In contrast, Japanese, Korean, and Navajo reverse the order of the verb (V) and the object (O). In other languages (e.g., Tagalog), the verb (V) precedes the subject (S) of the sentence.

The arrangement of the adjective (A) in relationship to the noun (N) is also presented for each language. In English, the adjective precedes the noun: red (A) dress (N); big (A) house (N). However, in languages such as French, Greek, Italian, and Vietnamese, the noun (N) precedes the adjective (A).

USE OF THE LANGUAGE DESCRIPTIONS

Some caution is necessary before using any of the language descriptions as a *standard* against which a child is compared. Each of the language descriptions represents a particular dialect. The language description for Spanish, for example, represents the language as it generally is used in Mexico. However, sizable portions of the Hispanic population in the United States also come from Puerto Rico, Cuba, and Central and South America. Moreover, many were born in the United States. Hence, the language descriptions may not be representative of the dialect spoken by an individual child. Dialect differences in the local community must be identified so that the language descriptions can be used appropriately.

Speech–language pathologists need to work closely with native speakers of the child's language to obtain information about phonemes that do not occur in English. By using the language descriptions and working with native speakers, one can begin to develop articulation tests in languages other than English. Word lists, for example, could be developed for use in screening children's production of particular speech sounds.

One cannot expect to conduct a comprehensive assessment of the child's speech and language functioning based solely on the information provided in the language descriptions. Additional references are needed, and one should also consult with speakers of the local dialect. The 15 language descriptions are presented in alphabetical order.

```
CANTONESE  [Chao 1969][Sino-Tibetan: Sinitic: South][S China
            (Canton); 27 million]

p pʰ    t̪ t̪ʰ      k kʰ kʷ kʰʷ    i         u  ī ȳ     ū   j w high falling
          cç cçh                e ø       o    ø̄             mid rising
f         ç            h            ɐ      ɛ̄        ɔ̄         mid level
m       n̪         ŋ                           ā              low falling
        l̪                                                     low rising
                                           CV(C)              low level

                                           non-phonemic stress

                                           SVO/AN
```

```
FRENCH (West Canadian) [Ellis 1965][Indo-European: Italic: Romance:
          Western][W Canada (British Columbia); 75 million]

p     t       k       i y   u
b     d       g       e ø ə o    ẽ ø̃   õ    j ɥ w    SVO/NA
f     s  ʃ            ɛ     ɔ    æ̃
v     z  ʒ            æ     ɑ
m     n  ɲ
      l
      r
```

GERMAN [Moulton 1962] [Indo-European: Germanic: West] [Germany; 100 million]

pʰ t̪ʰ kʰ i y u ī ȳ ū j w SVO/AN
b d̪ g e ø ə o ē ø̄ ō
pᶠ t̪ˢ [ɛ] ā
f s ʃ ç x h a
v z ʒ
m n̪
l̪
ʀ

GREEK (Modern) [Householder, Kazazis & Koutsoudas 1964] [Indo-European: Greek] [Greece; 8 million]

p t̪ k i u j phonemic stress
b d̪ g e o
tˢ a SVO/NA
dᶻ
f θ s x
v ð z ɣ
m n̪
l̪
ɾ

ITALIAN (Standard) [Agard & DiPietro 1969] [Indo-European: Italic: Romance: Western] [Italy; 60 million]

p p̄ t̪ t̪̄ k k̄ i u j w SVO/NA
b b̄ d̪ d̪̄ g ḡ e o
ɛ ɔ
t̪ˢ t̪̄ˢ č č̄ a
d̪ᶻ d̪̄ᶻ ǰ ǰ̄
f f̄ s̪ s̪̄ ʃ
v v̄
m m̄ n̪ n̪̄ ɲ
l̪ l̪̄ ʎ
ɾ̪ r̪

JAPANESE [Bloch 1950] [Altaic: Japanese] [Japan; 100 million]

p t̪ k i u j w high SOV/AN
b d̪ g e o low
t̪ˢ č a
ǰ
s ʃ h
z [ʒ]
m n̪ n̪̄
l
ɾ

KOREAN (Seoul) [Martin 1951] [Altaic:-] [Korea; 34 million]

p pʰ pˀ t̪ t̪ʰ t̪ˀ k kʰ kˀ i u ɯ ī ū ɯ̄ j w
č čʰ čˀ e [ø] o ɤ ē ō ɤ̄ non-phonemic stress
s sˀ h ɛ ɒ ɛ̄ ɒ̄
m n̪ ŋ SOV/AN
l

MANDARIN [Chao 1968] [Sino-Tibetan: Sinitic: North] [N China (Peking); 387 million]

p pʰ t̪ t̪ʰ k kʰ i y u j ɥ w high level
t̪ˢ t̪ˢʰ ṭˢ ṭˢʰ cᶜ cᶜʰ e o high rising
a low falling
f s̪ ṣ ç χ high falling
m n̪ ŋ
l̪ (C)V(C)
ɻ̣ [ʀ] SVO/AN phonemic stress

NAVAJO [Reichard 1951] [Na-Dene: Athapaskan-Eyak: Athapaskan] [Arizona; 120,000]

p t t^h $t^ʔ$ k k^h k^w $k^ʔ$ ʔ ɩ ɩ̄ ɩ̃ ɩ̃̄ j ^ʔj [w]
t^sh $t^{sʔ}$ t^l $t^{lʔ}$ čh $č^ʔ$ ɛ o ɛ̄ ō ɛ̃ õ ɛ̃̄ ȭ high
a ā ã ã̄ low
d^z d^l ǰ rising
s ʃ x x^w h falling
z ʒ ɣ $ɣ^w$
[m] ^ʔm n ^ʔn SOV/AN
l ɬ

POLISH (Warsaw) [Schenker 1973] [Indo-European: Slavic: West] [Poland; 35 million]

p p^j t̪ k k^j i u j w
b b^j d̪ g g^j ɛ ɔ [ɛ̃] ɔ̃ penultimate stress
a
$t̪^s$ č $c^ç$
$d̪^z$ ǰ $ɟ^j$ SVO/AN
f f^j s̪ ʃ ç x x^j
v v^j z̪ ʒ ʝ
m m^j n̪ ɲ
l
r

PORTUGUESE (Lisbon) [Head 1964] [Indo-European: Italic: Romance: West] [Portugal; 100 million]

p t̪ k i u ĩ ũ j w SVO/NA
b d̪ g e o ẽ õ
f s ʃ ɛ [ɐ] ɔ ɐ̃
v z̪ ʒ a
m n ɲ
l ʎ
ɾ R

SPANISH (Mexican) [Stockwell & Bowen 1965] [Indo-European: Italic: Romance: Western] [Mexico; 200 million]

p t̪ k i u j w phonemic stress
b d̪ g e o SVO/NA
č a
f s x
m n̪ ɲ
l
ɾ r

TAGALOG (Manila) [Schachter & Otanes 1972] [Austro-Tai: Austronesian: Indonesian: Hesperonesian: North Indonesian: Philippine] [Philippines; 10 million]

p t̪ k ʔ ɩ ɷ ɩ̄ ɷ̄ j w (C)CV(C)
b d̪ g e o ē ō non-phonemic stress
[č] ɐ ɐ̄
[f] s h VSO/AN~NA
m n̪ ŋ
l
ɾ

VIETNAMESE (Hanoi) [Thompson 1965] [Austro-Asíatic: Mon-Khmer: Viet-Muong] [Vietnam; 28 million]

p	t̪ʰ	t	c	k	ʔ	i		u		j w ɯ̯ ɒ̯
ɓ		ɗ							ɯ̌	
f	s̪			x	h	e		o	ɤ	
	z̪			ɣ		ɛ	ɐ	ɔ	ʌ	
m	n̪		ɲ	ŋ		æ				
	l̪									

high rising
high rising glottalized
higher mid trailing falling
low trailing
mid low dropping
low dropping

CV(C)(C)

SVO/NA

YIDDISH [Fal'kovich 1966] [Indo-European: Germanic: West] [E USSR; 4 million]

p	t̪		k		i		u	j
b	d̪		g		e		o	
						a		
	t̪ˢ	č						
f	s̪	ʃ	x					
v	z̪	ʒ		ɦ				
m	n̪							
	l̪							
	r̪		[ʀ]					

initial stress

SVO/AN

Appendix E

Exercises

EXERCISES

1. A researcher has developed a Spanish vocabulary test that was standardized on a national sample of 5000 Mexican American children. The researcher claims that the test is nonbiased and that the norms are valid for all Mexican American children. Prepare an argument to convince the researcher that bias exists in all tests.
2. A Japanese-speaking child is referred to you for testing. There are no teachers or instructional aides in your school district who speak the Japanese language. Develop a strategy for locating a Japanese-speaking adult in your community who can assist in the testing process. How would you go about training this individual?
3. Listed below are five sentences from a sentence imitation test developed by a speech–language pathologist who wishes to have the test translated into Spanish, Vietnamese, Korean, and numerous other languages. Your task is to help this speech–language pathologist by translating the five sentences below into at least one other language. Choose a language and develop a translation with the assistance of a native speaker. What problems did you encounter in developing appropriate translations?

   Sentences to be translated:
   1. My neighbor is running for mayor.
   2. The dog jumped.
   3. The boy has been chased by the dog several times.
   4. Neither the boy's ball nor the girl's ball has been taken from the box.
   5. The biggest child was second in line.
4. Construct an articulation screening test in a language that you do not speak, with the assistance of a native speaker of that language. What problems, if any, were encountered in the process?
5. The director of special education in your school district tells you that tests must never be administered to bilingual children by paraprofessionals. Prepare an argument to convince this individual that paraprofessionals can be used effectively.

6. You are asked to develop a standardized language test for use with the Vietnamese-speaking children in your school district. What steps would you take to develop an appropriate test instrument for these children?
7. Interview a bilingual adult from a non-Anglo culture. Find out about the culture, child-rearing practices, and attitudes towards the handicapped. What implications does the information obtained have for the assessment of children from this culture?

References

Adler, S. (1979). *Poverty children and their language*. New York: Grune & Stratton.

Albert, M. L., & Obler, L. K. (1978). *The bilingual brain*. New York: Academic Press.

Alexander, H. W. (1968). *An investigation of the cloze procedure as a measuring device designed to identify the independent, instruction, and frustration reading levels of pupils in the intermediate grades*. Unpublished doctoral dissertation, University of Illinois.

Alpiner, J., Ogden, J., & Wiggins, J. (1970). The utilization of supportive personnel in speech correction in the public schools: A pilot project. *Asha*, *12*, 599–604.

Anastasi, A. (1976). *Psychological testing*. New York: Macmillan.

Anderson, G. R., & Anderson, S. K. (1983). The exceptional Native American. In D. R. Omark & J. G. Erickson (Eds.), *The bilingual exceptual child*. San Diego: College-Hill Press.

Anderson, J. L. (1981). Considerations in phonological assessment. In J. G. Erickson and D. R. Omark (Eds.), *Communication assessment of the bilingual bicultural child*. Baltimore: University Park Press.

Anderson, M. P. (1983). Assessment personnel. In J. P. Gelatt & M. P. Anderson (Eds.), *Bilingual language learning system*. Rockville, MD: American Speech–Language–Hearing Association.

Austin, J. L. (1962). *How to do things with words*. London: Oxford University Press.

Bailey, D. B., & Harbin, G. L. (1980). Nondiscriminatory evaluation. *Exceptional Children*, *46*, 590–596.

Bates, E. (1976). *Language and context*. New York: Academic Press.

Bauman, R. (1971). An ethnographic framework of the investigation of communicative behaviors. *Asha*, *13*, 334–340.

Berringer, M. L. (1976). *The Ber-Sil Spanish Test*. Rancho Palos Verdes, CA: Ber-Sil Co.

Blackburn, J. (1983). Alternative 'immigration solution' offers promise. *Hispanic Link*, June 5.

Boehm, A. E. (1971). *The Boehm Test of Basic Concepts*. New York: Psychological Corporation.

Boone, D. R. (1971). *The voice and voice therapy*. Englewood Cliffs, NJ: Prentice–Hall.

Bormuth, J. R. (1962). *Cloze tests as measures of readability and comprehension ability*. Unpublished doctoral dissertation, Indiana University.

Bormuth, J. R. (1968). The cloze readability procedure. *Elementary English*, *45*, 429–436.

Briere, E. (1972). Are we really measuring proficiency with our foreign language tests? In B. Spolsky (Ed.), *The language education of minority children*. Rowley, MA: Newbury House.

Brigance, A. H. (1983). *Comprehensive Inventory of Basic Skills. North Billerica, MA: Curriculum Associates.*

Brigance, A. H. (1984). Assessment of Basic Skills: Spanish Edition. North Billerica, MA: Curriculum Associates.

Britton, L. P., & Britton, E. C. (1981). *Cultural traits of Asian students with implications for testing*. Sacramento: California State Department of Education.

Bronstein, A. (1973). Sociolinguistics, speech and language patterns. *Asha, 15*, 694–697.

Burt, M., & Dulay, H. (1978). Some guidelines for the assessment of oral language proficiency and dominance. *TESOL Quarterly, 12*, 177–191.

Burt, M., Dulay, H., & Hernandez-Chavez, E. (1976). *Bilingual Syntax Measure*. New York: Harcourt Brace Jovanovich.

Cairns, H. S., Cairns, C., & Williams, F. (1974). Some theoretical considerations of articulation substitution phenomena. *Language and Speech, 17*, 160–173.

California State Department of Education (1982). *A handbook for teaching Vietnamese-speaking students*. Los Angeles: Evaluation, Dissemination and Assessment Center, California State University.

Cancino, H., Rosansky, E. J., & Schumann, J. (1978). The acquisition of English negatives and interrogatives by native Spanish speakers. In E. M. Hatch (Ed.), *Second language acquisition*. Rowley, MA: Newbury House.

Carrier, J. (1970). A program of articulation therapy administered by mothers. *Journal of Speech and Hearing Disorders, 35*, 344–353.

Carrow, E. (1973). *Test for Auditory Comprehension of Language*. Hingham, MA: Teaching Resources.

Carrow, E. (1974).*Austin Spanish Articulation Test*. Hingham, MA: Teaching Resources.

Cazden, C. (1973). Cross-cultural biases in language tests. In J. W. Oller, Jr. & J. C. Richards (Eds.), *Focus on the learner*. Rowley, MA: Newbury House.

Cervantes, R. A. (1974). Problems and alternatives in testing Mexican American students. *Integrated Education, 12*, 33–37.

Chapman, R. S. (1981). Exploring children's communicative intents. In J. F. Miller (Ed.), *Assessing language production in children*. Baltimore: University Park Press.

Chomsky, N. (1965). *Aspects of the theory of syntax*. Cambridge, MA: MIT Press.

Cole, L., & Campbell-Calloway, M. (1983). Resource guide to multicultural tests and materials—Supplement 1. *Asha, 25*, 37–42.

Cole, L., & Snope, T. (1981). Resource guide to multicultural tests and materials. *Asha, 23*, 639–649.

Compton, A. J. (1970). Generative studies in children's phonological disorders. *Journal of Speech and Hearing Disorders, 35*, 315–339.

Cooper, J. C. (1983). Audiological screening and assessment of bilingual children. In D. R. Omark & J. G. Erickson (Eds.), *The bilingual exceptional child*. San Diego, CA: College-Hill Press.

Cornejo, R. (1973). The acquisition of lexicon in the speech of bilingual children. In P. Turner (Ed.), *Bilingualism in the southwest*. Tucson: University of Arizona Press.

Costello, J., & Bosler, S. (1976). Generalization and articulation instruction. *Journal of Speech and Hearing Disorders, 41*, 359–373.

Costello, J., & Schoen, J. (1978). The effectiveness of paraprofessionals and a speech clinician as agents of articulation intervention using programmed instruction. *Language, Speech, and Hearing Services in Schools, 9*, 118–128.

Cracker, H. V. (1971). *Clozentropy procedure as an instrument measuring oral English competencies of first grade children*. Unpublished doctoral dissertation, University of New Mexico.

Critchlow, D. E. (1974). *Dos Amigos Verbal Language Scales*. San Rafael, CA: Academic Therapy Publications.

Crystal, D., Fletcher, P., & Garman, M. (1976). *The grammatical analysis of language disability: A procedure for assessment and remediation*. New York: Elsevier-North Holland.

Cummins, J. (1981). The role of primary language development in promoting educational success for language minority students. In D. P. Dolson (Ed.), *Schooling and language minority students: A theoretical framework*. Los Angeles: Evaluation, Dissemination and Assessment Center, California State University.

Dale, P. (1977). Factors related to dysfluent speech in bilingual Cuban–American adolescents. *Journal of Fluency Disorders, 2*, 311–314.

Damico, J., & Oller, J. W., Jr. (1980). Pragmatic versus morphological/syntactic criteria for language referrals. *Language, Speech and Hearing Services in Schools, 11*, 85–94.

Damico, J. S., & Oller, J. W., Jr. (1984). *Spotting Language Problems*. San Diego: Los Amigos Research Associates.

Damico, J. S., Oller, J. W., Jr., & Storey, M. E. (1983). The diagnosis of language disorders in bilingual children: Surface-oriented and pragmatic criteria. *Journal of Speech and Hearing Disorders, 48*, 385–394.

Davis, H. (1970). Audiometry: Pure tone and simple speech tests. In H. Davis & S. R. Silverman (Eds.), *Hearing and deafness*. New York: Holt, Rinehart & Winston.

Day, E. C., McCollum, P. A., Cieslak, V. A., & Erickson, J. G. (1981). Discrete point testing of bilinguals: A review of selected tests. In J. G. Erickson & D. R. Omark (Eds.), *Communication assessment of the bilingual bicultural child*. Baltimore: University Park Press.

DeAvila, E., & Duncan, S. E. (1977). *Language Assessment Scales*. Corte Madero, CA: Linguametrics Group.

DeBlassie, R. R. (1980). *Testing Mexican American youth*. Hingham, MA: Teaching Resources.

DeBlassie, R. R., & Franco, J. N. (1983). Psychological and educational assessment of bilingual children. In D. R. Omark & J. G. Erickson (Eds.), *The bilingual exceptional child*. San Diego: College-Hill Press.

DeLeon Northrup, B. (1983). Audiological assessment. In J. P. Gelatt & M. P. Anderson (Eds.), *Bilingual language learning system*. Rockville, MD: American Speech-Language-Hearing Association.

Denich, B. S. (1970). Migration and network manipulation. In R. Spencer (Ed.), *Migration and anthropology*. Seattle: University of Washington Press.

Dickerson, L. J. (1974). *Internal and external patterning of phonological variability in the speech of Japanese learners of English: Toward a theory of second language acquisition*. Unpublished doctoral dissertation, University of Illinois.

Directory of bilingual speech–language pathologists and audiologists (1982). Rockville, MD: American Speech-Language-Hearing Association.

Dore, J. (1975). Holophrases, speech acts and language universals. *Journal of Child Language, 2*, 21–40.

Dore, J. (1978). Requestive systems in nursery school conversations: Analysis of talk in its social context. In R. Campbell & P. Smith (Eds.), *Recent advances in the psychology of language: Language development and mother–child interaction*. New York: Plenum Press.

Duffey, J. B., Salvia, J., Tucker, J., & Ysseldyke, J. (1981). Nonbiased assessment: A need for operationalism. *Exceptional Children*, *47*, 427–434.

Dulay, H., & Burt, M. (1973). Should we teach children syntax? *Language Learning*, *24*, 245–258.

Dulay, H., & Burt, M. (1974). Natural sequences in child second language acquisition. *Language Learning*, *24*, 37–53.

Dulay, H., & Burt, M. (1975). A new approach to discovering universals of child second language acquisition. In D. Dato (Ed.), *Developmental psycholinguistics*. Washington, DC: Georgetown University Press.

Dulay, H., Burt, M., & Krashen, S. (1982). *Language two*. New York: Oxford University Press.

Dulay, H., Hernandez-Chavez, E., & Burt, M. (1978). The process of becoming bilingual. In S. Singh & J. Lynch (Eds.), *Diagnostic procedures in hearing, speech and language*. Baltimore: University Park Press, 251–303.

Dunn, L. M., & Dunn, L. M. (1982). *Peabody Picture Vocabulary Test*. Circle Pines, MN: American Guidance Service.

Eames, E., & Goode, J. G. (1977). *Anthropology of the city*. Englewood Cliffs, NJ: Prentice–Hall.

Eibl-Eibesfeldt, I. (1975). *Ethology, the biology of behavior*. New York: Holt, Rinehart & Winston.

Eisenson, J. (1971). Aphasia in adults: Basic considerations. In L. E. Travis (Ed.), *Handbook of speech pathology and audiology*. Englewood Cliffs, NJ: Prentice–Hall.

Ekman, P. (1973). Cross-cultural studies of facial expression. In P. Ekman (Ed.), *Darwin and facial expression*. New York: Academic Press.

Ekman, P., & Friesen, W. (1975). *Unmasking the face*. Englewood Cliffs, NJ: Prentice–Hall.

Ekman, P., & Friesen, W. (1978). *The facial action coding system*. Palo Alto, CA: Consulting Psychologists Press.

Erickson, J. G. (1981). Communication assessment of the bilingual bicultural child: An overview. In J. G. Erickson & D. R. Omark (Eds.), *Communication assessment of the bilingual bicultural child*. Baltimore: University Park Press.

Erickson, J. G., & Omark, D. R. (1980). Social relationships and communicative interactions of mainstreamed communication handicapped preschool children. *Instructional Science*, *17*, 285–291.

Erickson, J. G., & Omark, D. R. (Eds.) (1981). *Communication assessment of the bilingual bicultural child*. Baltimore: University Park Press.

Erickson, J. G., & Walker, C. L. (1983). Bilingual exceptional children: What are the issues? In D. R. Omark & J. G. Erickson (Eds.), *The bilingual exceptional child*. San Diego: College-Hill Press.

Evard, B. L., & Sabers, D. L. (1979). Speech and language testing with distinct ethnic-racial groups: A survey of procedures for improving validity. *Journal of Speech and Hearing Disorders*, *44*, 271–281.

Fathman, A. (1975). Language background, age and the order of acquisition of English structures. In M. Burt & H. Dulay (Eds.), *New directions in second language learning, teaching, and bilingual education*. Washington, DC: TESOL.

Ferrer, O. (1960). Speech audiometry: A discrimination test for the Spanish language. *Laryngoscope*, *70*, 1541–1551.

Fisher, H. B., & Logemann, J. A. (1971). *Fisher-Logemann Test of Articulation Competence*. Boston: Houghton Mifflin.

Fishman, J. A. (1972). *Language in sociocultural change*. Stanford: Stanford University Press.

Frassinelli, L., Superior, K., & Meyers, J. (1983). A consultation model for speech and language intervention. *Asha*, *25*, 25–30.

Frith, G. H., & Teller, H. E. (1982). Using paraprofessionals in programs for hearing-impaired children. *Language, Speech, and Hearing Services in Schools*, *13*, 172–176.

Gamez-Huebner, M., Watson, D. L., & Omark, D. R. (1984). *Basic Elementary Skills Test—Spanish*. San Diego: Los Amigos Research Associates.

Garcia, E., Maez, G., & Gonzalez, G. (1981). A national study of Spanish/English bilingualism in young Hispanic children of the United States, *Bilingual Education Paper Series* (Vol. 4). Los Angeles: Evaluation, Dissemination and Assessment Center, California State University.

Gerken, K. G. (1978). Language dominance: A comparison of measures. *Language, Speech, and Hearing Services in Schools*, *9*, 187–196.

Gillis, M., & Weber, R. (1976). The emergence of sentence modalities in the English of Japanese-speaking children. *Language Learning*, *26*, 77–94.

Glass, L. (1979). Coping with the bilingual child. *Asha, 21*, 512–519.

Grant, J. (1983). The bilingual hearing impaired: Teaching children and preparing teachers. In D. R. Omark & J. G. Erickson (Eds.), *The bilingual exceptional child*. San Diego: College-Hill Press.

Graves, N., & Graves, T. (1974). Adaptive strategies in urban migration. In B. J. Siegel (Ed.), *Annual review of anthropology*. Guilford, CT: Dushkin Publishing Group.

Gronlund, N. E. (1981). *Measurement and evaluation in teaching*. New York: Macmillin.

Grossman, H. J. (Ed.) (1973). *Manual on terminology and classification in mental retardation*. Washington, DC: American Association on Mental Deficiency.

Grundin, H. U., Courtney, L., Langer, J., Pehrrson, H., Robinson, A., & Sakamoto, T. (1978). Cloze procedure and comprehension: An exploratory study across three languages. In D. Feitelson (Ed.), *Cross-cultural perspectives on reading and reading research*. Newark, DE: International Reading Association.

Hall, E. T. (1966). *The hidden dimension*. Garden City, NY: Doubleday.

Halliday, M. A. K. (1975). *Learning how to mean: Explorations in the development of language*. New York: Elsevier-North Holland.

Halliday, M. A. K. (1978). *Language as a social semiotic*. Baltimore: University Park Press.

Harris, G. (1982). Asha interviews Gail Harris, Indian advocate. *Asha*, *24*, 388–392.

Harris, M. (1975). *Comparison of individual and group instruction of parents in learning to administer an articulation program to their children*. Unpublished master's thesis, University of California, Santa Barbara.

Hernandez-Chavez, E. (1972). *Early code separation in the second language speech of Spanish-speaking children*. Paper presented at the Stanford Child Language Research Forum, Stanford University, Stanford, CA.

Hersey, P., & Blanchard, K. H. (1977). *Management of organizational behavior: Utilizing human resources*. Englewood Cliffs, NJ: Prentice–Hall.

Hittleman, D. R. (1978). *Developmental reading: A psycholinguistic perspective*. Chicago: Rand McNally.

Hodson, B. W., Diamond, F., Meza, P., & Cornejo, R. (1983). *Phonological analysis of Spanish utterances of Mexican-American children*. Paper presented at the Convention of the American Speech–Language–Hearing Association, Cincinnati, OH.

Hodson, B. W., & Paden, E. P. (1983). *Targeting intelligible speech*. San Diego: College-Hill Press.

Hresko, W. P., Reid, D. K., & Hammill, D. D. (1981). *The Test of Early Language Development*. Austin: Pro-Ed.

Hresko, W. P., Reid, D. K., & Hammill, D. D. (1982). *Prueba del Desarrollo Inicial del Lenguaje*. Austin: Pro-Ed.

Hymes, D. (1971). Sociolinguistics and the ethnography of speaking. In E. Ardenar (Ed.), *Social anthropology and language*. London: Tavistock.

Hymes, D. (1974). *Foundations in sociolinguistics*. Philadelphia: University of Pennsylvania Press.

Iglesias, A. (1983). Phonology. In J. P. Gelatt & M. P. Anderson (Eds.), *Bilingual language learning system*. Rockville, MD: American Speech–Language–Hearing Association.

Ingram, D. (1976). *Phonological disability in children*. New York: Elsevier.

James, P. (1974). *James Language Dominance Test*. Hingham, MA: Teaching Resources.

Juarez, M. (1983). Assessment and treatment of minority-language-handicapped children: The role of the monolingual speech–language pathologist. *Topics in Language Disorders*, *3*, 57–66.

Kachru, B. B. (1965). The Indianness of Indian English. *Word*, *21*, 391–410.

Kaufman, R. A. (1972). *Educational system planning*. Englewood Cliffs, NJ: Prentice–Hall.

Keenan, J. S., & Brassell, E. G. (1975). *Aphasia Language Performance Scales*. Murfressboro, TN: Pinnacle Press.

Kincheloe, S. (1970). Churches and cities change together. In H. M. Hughes (Ed.), *Cities and city life*. Boston: Allyn & Bacon.

Kleiner, R., & Parker, S. (1975). Network participation and psychosocial impairment in an urban environment. In H. Meadows & E. Mizruchi (Eds.), *Urbanism, urbanization and change*. Reading, MA: Addison–Wesley.

Klima, E. S., & Bellugi, U. (1966). Syntactic regularities in the speech of children. In J. Lyons & R. Wales (Eds.), *Psycholinguistic papers* (pp. 183–219). Edinburgh: Edinburgh University Press.

Krashen, S., Long, M. A., & Scarcella, R. C. (1979). Age, rate and eventual attainment in second language acquisition. *TESOL Quarterly*, *13*, 521–534.

Labov, W. (1971). The study of language in its social context. In J. A. Fishman (Ed.), *Advances in the sociology of language*. The Hague: Mouton.

Laila Khan, L. M. (1982). A review of 16 major phonological processes. *Language, Speech, and Hearing Services in Schools*, *13*, 77–85.

Langdon, H. W. (1983). Assessment and intervention strategies for the bilingual language-disordered student. *Exceptional Children*, *50*, 37–46.

Lee, L. (1974). *Developmental sentence analysis*. Evanston, IL: Northwestern University Press.

Leeman, E. M. (1981). Evaluating language assessment tests: Some practical considerations. In J. G. Erickson & D. R. Omark (Eds.), *Communication assessment of the bilingual child*. Baltimore: University Park Press.

Lemert, E. M. (1962). Stuttering and social structure in two pacific societies. *Journal of Speech and Hearing Disorders*, *27*, 3–10.

Leonard, L., Prutting, C., Perozzi, J. A., & Berkley, R. K. (1978). Non-standardized approaches to the assessment of language behaviors. *Asha*, *20*, 371–379.

Leonard, L. B., & Weiss, A. L. (1983). Application of nonstandardized assessment procedures to diverse linguistic populations. *Topics in Language Disorders*, *3*, 35–45.

Lerner, J. W. (1976). *Children with learning disabilities*. Boston: Houghton Mifflin.

Linares, N. (1981). Rules for calculating mean length of utterance in morphemes for Spanish. In J. G. Erickson & D. R. Omark (Eds.), *Communication assessment of the bilingual bicultural child*. Baltimore: University Park Press.

Linares, N. (1983). Management of communicatively handicapped Hispanic American children. In D. R. Omark & J. G. Erickson (Eds.), *The bilingual exceptional child*. San Diego: College-Hill Press.

Locke, L. (1981). Issues and procedures in the analysis of syntax and semantics. In J. G. Erickson & D. R. Omark (Eds.), *Communication assessment of the bilingual bicultural child*. Baltimore: University Park Press.

Lombardino, L., & Mangan, N. (1983) Parents as language trainers: Language programming with developmentally delayed children. *Exceptional Children*, *49*, 358–361.

Lucas, E. V. (1980). *Semantic and pragmatic language disorders*. Rockville, MD: Aspen Systems Corporation.

Makino, T. (1979). *English morpheme acquisition order of Japanese secondary school students*. Unpublished doctoral dissertation, University of New Mexico.

Mares, S. (1980). *Pruebas de expressión oral y percepción de la lengua española*. Downey, CA: Office of the Los Angeles County Superintendent of Schools.

Martin, F. N., & Hart, D. B. (1978). Measurement of speech thresholds of Spanish-speaking children by non-Spanish clinicians. *Journal of Speech and Hearing Disorders*, *43*, 255–262.

Mason, M. A., Smith, B. F., & Henshaw, M. M. (1976). *La "Meda": Medida Española de Articulación*. San Ysidro, CA: San Ysidro School District.

Matluck, J., & Mace, B. (1973). Language characteristics of Mexican-American children: Implications for assessment. *Journal of School Psychology*, *2*, 365–386.

Mattes, L. J. (1976). *Grammatical responses of adult aphasics on structured experimental tasks and in spontaneous speech: A comparison*. Unpublished master's thesis, University of California, Santa Barbara.

Mattes, L. J. (1982a). *Classroom oral language development: An elementary school oral language curriculum*. Springfield, IL: Thomas.

Mattes, L. J. (1982b). The elicited language analysis procedure: A method for scoring sentence imitation tasks. *Language, Speech, and Hearing Services in Schools*, *13*, 37–41.

Mattes, L. J. (1982c). *The identification of Spanish-speaking children with speech and language handicaps: An analysis of current assessment practices in speech and language therapy programs with proposed assessment guidelines*. Unpublished doctoral dissertation, University of San Diego.

Mattes, L. J. (1984). *Spanish Language Assessment Procedures: A Communication Skills Inventory*. Oceanside, CA: Academic Communication Associates.

McCollum, P. A. (1981). Concepts in bilingualism and their relationship to language assessment. In J. G. Erickson & D. R. Omark (Eds.), *Communication assessment of the bilingual bicultural child*. Baltimore: University Park Press.

McCollum, P. A., & Day, E. C. (1981). Quasi-integrative approaches: Discrete point scoring of expressive language samples. In J. G. Erickson & D. R. Omark (Eds.), *Communication assessment of the bilingual bicultural child*. Baltimore: University Park Press.

McDermott, R. P. (1977). The ethnography of speaking and reading. In R. W. Shuy (Ed.), *Linguistic theory: What can it say about reading*. Newark, DE: International Reading Association.

McReynolds, L. V., & Elbert, M. (1981). Criteria for phonological process analysis. *Journal of Speech and Hearing Disorders*, *46*, 197–204.

Mehrabian, A. (1972). *Nonverbal communication*. Chicago: Aldine-Atherton.

Mercer, J. R. (1979). *SOMPA: System of Multicultural Pluralistic Assessment*. New York: Psychological Corporation.

Mercer, J. R. (1980). Testing and assessment practices in multiethnic education. In J. Banks & B. Shin (Eds.), *Education in the 80's: Multiethnic education*. Washington, DC: National Education Association.

Mercer, J. R. (1983). Issues in the diagnosis of language disorders in students whose primary language is not English. *Topics in Language Disorders*, *3*, 46–56.

Meyen, E. L. (1978). *Exceptional children and youth*. Denver: Love.

Meyerson, M. D. (1983). Genetic counseling for families of Chicano children. In D. R. Omark & J. G. Erickson (Eds.), *The bilingual exceptional child*. San Diego: College-Hill Press.

Miller, J. F. (1981). *Assessing language production in children*. Baltimore: University Park Press.

Milon, J. (1974). The development of negation in English by a second language learner. *TESOL Quarterly*, *8*, 137–143.

Moncada, L. R., & Marshall, M. H. (1982). Examenes para Diagnosticar Impedimentos de Afasia. Murfreesboro, TN: Pinnacle Press.

Moncur, J. P., & Brackett, I. P. (1974). *Modifying vocal behavior*. New York: Harper & Row.

Muma, J. R. (1978). *Language handbook*. Englewood Cliffs, NJ: Prentice–Hall.

Newcomer, P. L., & Hammill, D. D. (1982). *Test of Language Development*. Austin: Pro-Ed.

Nutter, B. L. (1974). *Presentation methods, deletion patterns and passage types for use with aural cloze*. Unpublished doctoral dissertation, University of Arizona.

Oakland, T., & Laosa, L. M. (1977). Professional, legislative, and judicial influences on psychoeducational assessment practices in schools. In T. Oakland (Ed.), *Psychological and educational assessment of minority children*. New York: Brunner/Mazel.

O'Brien, C. A. (1973). *Teaching the language-different child to read*. Columbus: Merrill.

Oller, J. W., Jr. (1979). *Language tests at school*. London: Longman.

Oller, J. W., Jr. (1983). Testing proficiences and diagnosing language disorders in bilingual children. In D. R. Omark & J. G. Erickson (Eds.), *The bilingual exceptional child*. San Diego: College-Hill Press.

Oller, J. W., Jr., Bowen, J. D., Dien, T. T., & Mason, V. W. (1972). Cloze tests in English, Thai, and Vietnamese: Native and non-native performance. *Language Learning, 22*, 1–15.

Omark, D. R. (1981a). Conceptualizations of bilingual children: Testing the norm. In J. G. Erickson & D. R. Omark (Eds.), *Communication assessment of the bilingual bicultural child*. Baltimore: University Park Press.

Omark, D. R. (1981b). Pragmatics and ethological techniques for the observational assessment of children's communicative abilities. In J. G. Erickson & D. R. Omark (Eds.), *Communication assessment of the bilingual bicultural child*. Baltimore: University Park Press.

Omark, D. R., & Watson, D. L. (1983a). *Assessing bilingual exceptional children: In-service manual*. San Diego: Los Amigo Research Associates.

Omark, D. R., & Watson, D. L. (1983b). Psychological testing and bilingual education: The need for reconceptualization. In D. R. Omark & J. G. Erickson (Eds.), *The bilingual exceptional child*. San Diego: College-Hill Press.

Ortiz, de R. (1980). The acquisition of Spanish as a native language. In H. Dulay, M. Burt, & D. McKeon (Eds.), *Testing and teaching communicatively handicapped children*. Sacramento: California State Department of Education.

Pacheco, R., & Omark, D. R. (1984). *Special education and bilingual education: Working together*. San Diego: College-Hill Press.

Page, W. D. (1977). Comprehension and cloze performance. *Reading World, 17*, 1–12.

Perkins, W. H. (1971). *Speech pathology: An applied behavioral science*. St. Louis: Mosby.

Perrone, P. A., & Aleman, N. (1983). Educating the talented child in a pluralistic society. In D. R. Omark & J. G. Erickson (Eds.), *The bilingual exceptional child*. San Diego: College-Hill Press.

Pickering, M. (1976). Bilingual/bicultural education and the speech pathologist. *Asha, 18*, 175–179.

Pickett, A. L. (1979). Paraprofessionals in special education: The state of the art—1979. New York: National Resource Center for Paraprofessionals in Special Education, New Careers Training Laboratory, Center for Advanced Study in Education, City University of New York.

Porch, B. (1967). *Porch Index of Communicative Ability*. Palo Alto, CA: Consulting Psychologists Press.

Prather, E. M., Hedrick, D. L., & Kern, C. A. (1975). Articulation development in children aged two to four years. *Journal of Speech and Hearing Disorders, 40*, 179–191.

Prutting, C. A. (1982). Pragmatics as social competence. *Journal of Speech and Hearing Disorders, 47*, 123–134.

Prutting, C. A. (1983). Assessing communicative behavior using a language sample. In D. R. Omark & J. G. Erickson (Eds.), *The bilingual exceptional child*. San Diego: College-Hill Press.

Prutting, C. A., & Connolly, J. E. (1976). Imitation: A closer look. *Journal of Speech and Hearing Disorders, 41*, 412–422.

Public Law 94-142 (1975, November 19). Education for All Handicapped Children Act.

Ravem, R. (1968). Language acquisition in a second language environment. *International Review of Applied Linguistics, 6*, 175–185.

Reynolds, M. C. (1962). A framework for considering some issues in special education. *Exceptional Children, 28*, 367–370.

Reynolds, M. C., & Birch, J. W. (1982). *Teaching exceptional children in all America's schools*. Reston, VA: Council for Exceptional Children.

Roberts, B. (1974). *Organizing strangers*. Austin: University of Texas Press.

Rosansky, E. J. (1976). Methods and morphemes in second language acquisition research. *Language Learning, 26*, 409–425.

Rueda, R., & Perozzi, J. A. (1977). Comparison of two Spanish tests of receptive language. *Journal of Speech and Hearing Disorders, 42*, 210–215.

Ruhlen, N. (1976). *Guide to the languages of the world*. San Diego: Los Amigo Research Associates (distributor).

Scalero, A., & Eskenazi, C. (1976). The use of supportive personnel in a public school speech and language program. *Language, Speech, and Hearing Services in Schools, 7*, 150–158.

Scholz, G. D., Hendricks, D., Spurling, R., Johnson, M., & Vandenburg, L. (1980). Is language ability divisible or unitary? A factor analysis of twenty-two language proficiency tests. In J. W. Oller, Jr. & K. Perkins (Eds.), *Research in language testing*. Rowley, MA: Newbury House.

Schuell, H. (1965). *The Minnesota Test for Differential Diagnosis of Aphasia*. Minneapolis: University of Minnesota Press.

Searle, J. R. (1969). Speech acts: An essay in the philosophy of language. Cambridge: Cambridge University Press.

Silverman, R. J., Noa, J. K., & Russell, R. H. (1976). *Oral language tests for bilingual students: An evaluation of language dominance and proficiency instruments*. Portland: Northwest Regional Educational Laboratory.

Silverman, S. R. (1971). The education of deaf children. In L. E. Travis (Ed.), *Handbook of speech pathology and audiology*. Englewood Cliffs, NJ: Prentice–Hall.

Skoczylas, R. V. (1971). *Home Bilingual Usage Estimate*. 7649 Santa Inez Ct., Gilroy, Ca 95020.

Skuttnabb-Kangas, T., & Toukomaa, P. (1976). *Teaching migrant children's mother tongue and learning the language of the host country in the context of the sociocultural situation of the migrant family*. Helsinki: Finnish National Commission for UNESCO.

Sommer, R. (1969). *Personal space*. Englewood Cliffs, NJ: Prentice–Hall.

Sridhar, K. K. (1981). Pragmatics and language assessment. In J. G. Erickson & D. R. Omark (Eds.), *Communication assessment of the bilingual bicultural child*. Baltimore: University Park Press.

Stevenson, D. (1974). *A preliminary investigation of construct validity and the Test of English as a Foreign Language*. Unpublished doctoral dissertation, University of New Mexico.

Stewart, J. L. (1960, April). The problem of stuttering in certain North American Indian societies. *Journal of Speech and Hearing Disorders*. Monograph Supplement 6.

Stewart, J. L. (1983). Communication disorders in the American Indian population. In D. R. Omark & J. G. Erickson (Eds.), *The bilingual exceptional child*. San Diego: College-Hill Press.

Stockwell, R. P., & Bowen, J. D. (1965). *The sounds of English and Spanish*. Chicago: University of Chicago Press.

Taylor, O. T., & Payne, K. T. (1983). Culturally valid testing: A proactive approach. *Topics in Language Disorders, 3*, 1–7.

Teitelbaum, B. (1977). *The validity of various techniques measuring children's bilingualism*. Arlington, VA: ERIC Document Reproduction Service No. ED 140 665. Reprinted from Bilingual Education Project, Ontario Institute for Studies in Education, Ontario, Canada.

Templin, M. C., & Darley, F. L. (1960). *The Templin–Darley Tests of Articulation*. Iowa City: State University of Iowa.

Tewksbury, G. (1948). *Speak Chinese*. New Haven, CN: Far Eastern Publications, Yale University.

Tolliver-Weddington, G., & Meyerson, M. D. (1983). Training paraprofessionals for identification and intervention with communicatively disordered bilinguals. In D. R. Omark & J. G. Erickson (Eds.), *The bilingual exceptional child*. San Diego: College-Hill Press.

Toronto, A. S. (1972). *Southwestern Spanish Articulation Test*. Austin: National Education Laboratory Publishers.

Toronto, A. S. (1973). *Screening Test of Spanish Grammar*. Evanston, IL: Northwestern University Press.

Toronto, A. S. (1976). Developmental assessment of Spanish grammar. *Journal of Speech and Hearing Disorders, 41*, 150–171.

Toronto, A. S., Leverman, D., Hanna, C., Rosenzweig, P., & Maldonado, A. (1975). *Del Rio Language Screening Test*. Austin: National Educational Laboratory.

Toronto, A. S., & Merrill, S. (1983). Developing local normed assessment instruments. In D. R. Omark & J. G. Erickson (Eds.), *The bilingual exceptional child*. San Diego: College-Hill Press.

Tough, J. (1977). *The development of meaning*. New York: Halsted Press.

Trotter, R. J. (1974). Cities, crowding and crime. *Science News, 106*, 282–283.

Tyack, D., & Gottsleben, R. (1974). *Language sampling, analysis and training*. Palo Alto, CA: Consulting Psychologists Press.

Van Riper, C. (1972). *Speech correction: Principles and methods*. Englewood Cliffs, NJ: Prentice–Hall.

Vaughn-Cooke, F. (1983). Improving language assessment in minority children. *Asha, 25*, 29–34.

Wallis, C. (1983, June 6). Stress: Can we cope? *Time*.

Walters, J. (1979). Language variation in assessing bilingual children's communicative competence. *Bilingual Education Paper Series* (Vol. 3). Los Angeles: Evaluation, Dissemination and Assessment Center, California State University.

Walters, J. (1981). The role of contextual factors in language use and language assessment. In J. G. Erickson & D. R. Omark (Eds.), *Communication assessment of the bilingual bicultural child*. Baltimore: University Park Press.

Wardhaugh, R. (1970). The contrastive analysis hypothesis. *TESOL Quarterly, 4*, 123–130.

Watson, D. L., Grouell, S. L., Heller, B., & Omark, D. R. (1981). *Nondiscriminatory assessment: Test matrix* (Vol. 2). San Diego: Los Amigos Research Associates.

Watson, D. L., Omark, D. R., Grouell, S., & Heller, B. (1981). *Nondiscriminatory assessment: A practitioner's guide* (Vol. I). San Diego: Los Amigos Research Associates.

Wei, T. T. D. (1983). The Vietnamese refugee child: Understanding cultural differences. In D. R. Omark & J. G. Erickson (Eds.), *The bilingual exceptional child.* San Diego: College-Hill Press.

Weiner, F. F. (1979). *Phonological process analysis.* Baltimore: University Park Press.

Weiss, C. E. (1978). *Weiss Comprehensive Articulation Test.* Hingham, MA: Teaching Resources.

Wepman, J. M., & Jones, L. V. (1961). *Studies in aphasia: An approach to testing.* Chicago: Education Industry Service.

West, R., & Ansberry, M. (1968). *The rehabilitation of speech.* New York: Harper & Row.

Woodcock, R. W. (1982). *Woodcock Spanish Psycho-Educational Battery.* Hingham, MA: Teaching Resources.

Woodcock, R. W. (1982). *Woodcock Language Proficiency Battery (Spanish form). Hingham, MA: Teaching Resources.*

Woodcock, R. W., & Johnson, M. B. (1977). *Woodcock-Johnson Psycho-Educational Battery.* Hingham, MA: Teaching Resources.

Yasuda, A. (1970). Articulatory skills in three year old children. *Studia Phonologica, 5,* 52–71.

AUTHOR INDEX

A

Alder, S., 11
Albert, M. L., 63
Aleman, N., 50
Alexander, H. W., 86
Alpiner, J., 31
Anastasi, A., 96
Anderson, G. R., 45, 46
Anderson, J. L., 5–6
Anderson, M. P., 32
Anderson, S. K., 45, 46
Ansberry, M., 12
Austin, J. L., 77

B

Bailey, D. B., 65, 98
Bates, E., 51, 73, 75
Bauman, R., 45
Bellugi, U., 8
Beringer, M. L., 120
Berkley, R. K., 72
Birch, J. W., 46
Blackburn, J., 43
Blanchard, K. H., 30
Boehm, A. E., 60, 121
Boone, D. R., 3
Bormuth, J. R., 86
Bosler, S., 31
Bowen, J. D., 6, 86
Brackett, I. P., 3
Brassell, E. G., 62
Briere, E., 58, 75
Brigance, A. H., 84, 117, 119
Britton, E. C., 91
Britton, L. P., 91
Bronstein, A., 68
Burt, M., 5, 6, 8, 54–55, 59, 66, 120

C

Cairns, C., 5
Cairns, H. S., 5
California State Department of Education, 44
Campbell-Calloway, 113
Cancino, H., 8
Carrier, J., 31
Carrow, E., 53, 59, 119
Cazden, C., 58
Cervantes, R. A., 66
Chapman, R. S., 78
Chomsky, N., 51
Cieslak, V. A., 52
Cole, L., 113
Compton, A. J., 94
Connolly, J. E., 84
Cooper, J. C., 64, 65
Cornejo, R., 5, 94
Costello, J., 31, 109
Courtney, L., 86
Cracker, H. V., 87
Critchlow, D. E., 121
Crystal, D., 82
Cummins, J., 55, 104

D

Dale, P., 4
Damico, J. S., 23, 81
Darley, F. L., 53

Davis, H., 64
Day, E. C., 52, 59, 60, 113
DeAvila, E., 55, 85, 122
DeBlassie, R. R., 54, 58
DeLeon Northrup, B., 64
Denich, B. S., 43
Diamond, F., 94
Dickerson, L. J., 5
Dien, T. T., 86
Dore, J., 77
Duffey, J. B., 65, 98
Dulay, H., 5, 6, 8, 10, 11, 54–55, 59, 66, 120
Duncan, S. E., 55, 85, 122
Dunn, Leota M., 90, 98
Dunn, Lloyd M., 90, 98

E

Eames, E., 47
Eibl-Eiblesfeldt, I., 73
Eisenson, J., 62
Ekman, P., 11, 73
Elbert, M., 4
Erickson, J. G., 51, 52, 56, 65, 73, 79, 107, 131
Eskenazi, C., 31
Evard, B. L., 67

F

Fathman, A., 8
Ferrer, O., 64
Fisher, H. B., 53
Fishman, J. A., 11
Fletcher, P., 82
Franco, J. N., 58
Frassinelli, L., 108
Friesen, W., 73
Frith, G. H., 31, 32

G

Gamez-Huebner, M., 96
Garcia, E., 82
Garman, M., 82
Gerken, H. G., 55
Gillis, M., 8
Glass, L., 27
Gonzalez, G., 82
Goode, J. G., 43
Gottsleben, R., 74, 82
Grant, J., 12, 107
Graves, N., 43
Graves, T., 43
Gronlund, N. E., 97
Grossman, H. J., 82
Grouell, S. L., 49, 55, 61, 67, 68, 97, 113
Grundin, H. V., 86

H

Hall, E. T., 11
Halliday, M. A. K., 11, 77
Hammill, D. D., 61, 97, 98, 113, 114
Hanna, C., 61, 121
Harbin, G. L., 65, 98
Harris, G., 45
Harris, M., 31, 109
Hart, D. B., 64
Hedrick, D. L., 93
Heller, B., 49, 55, 61, 67, 68, 97, 113
Hendricks, D., 87
Henshaw, M. M., 53, 123
Hernandez-Chavez, 6, 9, 54–55, 120
Hersey, P., 30
Hittleman, D. R., 86
Hodson, B. W., 4, 54, 94
Hresko, W. P., 61, 113, 114, 119
Hymes, D., 11, 44

I

Iglesias, A., 53
Ingram, D., 54

J

James, P., 54
Johnson, M., 87
Johnson, M. B., 116
Jones, L. V., 62
Juarez, M., 7, 39, 104

K

Kachru, B. B., 2
Kaufman, R. A., 19
Keenan, J. S., 62
Kern, C. A., 93
Kincheloe, S., 42
Kleiner, R., 44
Klima, E. S., 8
Krashen, S., 5, 104

L

Labov, W., 77
Laila Khan, L. M., 94
Langdon, H. W., 23, 106
Langer, J., 86
Laosa, L. M., 1, 4
Lee, L., 74, 82
Leeman, E. M., 58
Lemert, E. M., 4
Leonard, L., 72, 88, 98
Lerner, J. W., 110
Leverman, D., 61, 121
Linares, N., 2, 82
Locke, L., 5
Logemann, J. A., 53
Lombardino, L., 108
Long, M. A., 194
Lucas, E. V., 77, 100

M

Mace, B., 5
Maez, G., 82
Makino, T., 8
Maldonado, A., 61, 121
Mangan, N., 108
Mares, S., 61, 114, 119
Marshall, M. H., 62, 122
Martin, F. N., 64
Mason, M. A., 53, 123
Mason, V. W., 86
Matluck, J., 5
Mattes, L. J., 14, 31, 53, 57, 63, 79, 84, 85, 91, 100, 107, 124
McCollum, P. A., 2, 52, 113
McDermott, R. P., 11
McReynolds, L. V., 4
Mehrabian, A., 11
Mercer, J. R., 1, 71, 82
Merrill, S., 61, 89, 95
Meyen, E. L., 104
Meyers, J., 108
Meyerson, M. D., 38, 39
Meza, P., 94
Miller, J. F., 12, 74, 83
Milon, J., 8
Moncada, L. R., 62, 122
Moncur, J. P., 3
Muma, J. R., 74

N

Newcomer, P. L., 97, 98
Noa, J. K., 55
Nutter, B. L., 87

O

Oakland, T., 1
Obler, L. K., 63
O'Brien, C. A., 5
Ogden, J., 31
Oller, J. W., Jr., 23, 52, 81, 86, 87
Omark, D. R., 49, 55, 56, 57, 61, 67, 68, 73, 79, 94, 97, 106, 113
Ortiz, R., 66

P

Pacheco, R., 106
Paden, E. P., 4, 54, 94
Page, W. D., 86
Parker, S., 44
Payne, K. T., 71
Pehrrson, H., 86
Perkins, W. H., 2
Perozzi, J. A., 59
Perrone, P. A., 50
Pickering, M., 107
Pickett, A. L., 31
Porch, B., 62
Prather, E. M., 93
Prutting, C., 13, 52, 72, 74, 84

R

Ravem, R., 8
Reid, D. K., 61, 113, 114
Reynolds, M. C., 46
Roberts, B., 44
Robinson, A., 86
Rosansky, E. J., 8
Rosenzweig, P., 61, 121
Rueda, R., 59
Ruhlen, N., 93, 131
Russell, R. H., 55

S

Sabers, D. L., 67
Sakamoto, T., 86
Salvia, J., 65
Scalero, A., 31
Scarcella, R. C., 104
Schoen, J., 31, 109
Scholz, G. D., 87
Schuell, H., 62
Schumann, J., 8
Searle, J. R., 77
Silverman, R. J., 55
Silverman, S. R., 12
Skoczylas, R. V., 56
Skuttnabb-Kangas, T., 104
Smith, B. F., 53, 123
Snope, T., 113
Sommer, R., 11
Spurling, R., 87
Sridhar, K. K., 75
Stevenson, D., 87
Stewart, J. L., 4, 65
Stockwell, R. P., 6
Storey, M. E., 23, 81
Superior, K., 108

T

Taylor, O. T., 71
Teitelbaum, B., 56
Teller, H. E., 31, 32
Templin, M. C., 53
Tewksbury, G., 90
Tolliver-Weddington, G., 39
Toronto, A. S., 53, 61, 82, 89, 95, 121, 123, 125
Tough, J., 78
Toukomaa, P., 104
Trotter, R. J., 44
Tucker, J., 65
Tyack, D., 74, 82

V

Vandenberg, L., 87
Van Riper, C., 3, 4
Vaughn-Cooke, F., 71, 72, 91, 92, 99

W

Walker, C. L., 107, 131
Wallis, C., 44
Walters, J., 56, 75
Wardhaugh, R., 5
Watson, D. L., 48, 55, 61, 67, 68, 73, 96, 97, 113
Weber, R., 8
Wei, T. T. D., 44, 45, 81
Weiner, F. F., 54
Weiss, A. L., 72
Weiss, C. E., 53
Wepman, J. M., 62
West, R., 12
Wiggins, J., 31
Williams, F., 31
Woodcock, R. W., 115, 116, 119

Y

Yasuda, A., 93
Ysseldyke, J., 65

SUBJECT INDEX

A

Adaptive behavior measures, 81–82
Adaptive Behavior Inventory for Children, 82
Adaptive Behavior Scale, 82
American Speech-Language Hearing Association, 25, 33, 34
Anthropological assessment technique, 41
Aphasia Language Performance Scales, 62
Aphasia
  definition of, 62
  tests, 62–63
Apraxia, 62
Articulation
  differences, 4–6
  disorders, 2, 4–7
  tests, 23, 52–54
    development of, 93–95
  See also Phonological development
Assessment instruments
  administration of, 67–68
  construction of, 67, 93–101
  interpretation of, 29, 68–70, 100
  modification of, 63, 67, 81, 91–93
  reviewing results of, 26–29
  selection of, 65–67
  using scores from, 1, 68–70
  See also Tests
Assessment personnel
  selection of, 25–26, 36
  training of, 17–18, 21–22, 23, 25, 29, 30, 35–39
Audiological assessment, 12–13, 64–65
Austin Spanish Articulation Test, 53, 119–120

B

Behavioral Inventory of Speech Act Performances, 100
Ber-Sil Spanish Test, 120
Bias in assessment, 1, 65
  elimination of, 1, 14–15, 71
Bilingual special education programs, 106–107
Bilingual Oral Language Development (BOLD), 79–80
Bilingual
  definition of, 2
Bilingual program specialists, 29–30
Bilingual Syntax Measure, 8, 54–55, 120
Boehm Test of Basic Concepts, 60, 121
Borrowing, *see* Linguistic borrowing
BRIGANCE® Assessment of Basic Skills, 117–118

C

Case history, 9, 14, 46–49, 63
Checklists, *see* Inventories for communication assessment
Child-rearing practices, 47
Cloze procedure, 86–87
Code of Ethics, 33, 34
Code switching, 10–11, 63
Communicative competence
  pragmatics and, 51, 75–77
  testing, 11, 51–52, 56, 75, 77–78
  See also Functional language use

Communicative differences
versus disorders, 1–15, 18, 30
See also Language
Communication samples, *see* Samples of natural communication
Communication style, 77
Community resources, 18, 21, 24–25
Comprehension of Oral Language Test, 55
Comprehensive Inventory of Basic Skills, 84
Consultation model, 108–109
Contextual factors, 11–12, 72
communication sampling and, 74–76
effect of, 10, 27, 69, 81
Contrastive analysis, 5–6
Core inventory of phonemes, 93–94
Court cases, *see* Litigation
Criterion-referenced tests, 13, 61, 84–85, 117–118
construction of, 98–100
limitations of, 119
Cultural attitudes
toward education, 45, 50
toward handicaps, 4, 38, 45–46
Cultural differences, 1, 4, 11, 77, 103, 107
and functional language use, 11, 72–73, 99
and test performance, 17, 27, 57–58, 60, 66, 68, 91–92
Cultural heritage
maintenance of, 50
Cultural norms, 72, 78

D

Del Rio Language Screening Test, 57, 61, 121
Developmental Assessment of Spanish Grammar, 82
Developmental errors, 7–9
Developmental Sentence Scoring, 82
Dialect differences, 15
and test performance, 53, 61, 66
Discourse rules, 11, 73, 78
Discrete point tests, 51–52, 60
definition of, 51
use of, 52
weaknesses of, 52–56
Dos Amigos Verbal Language Scales, 55, 121–122

E

Education for All Handicapped Children Act, *see* Public Law 94-142
Elicited Language Analysis Procedure, 84
Elicited language production tasks, 83–85, 99–100
English language proficiency tests, 56–58
Environmental influences, 41–45, 47–50
See also Language environment
Ethical issues
and use of paraprofessionals, 32–33
Examines para Diagnosticar Impedimentos de Afasia, 62, 122

F

Family structure
role of members, 44
size, 44, 47
Fisher-Logemann Test of Articulation Competence, 53
Fluency disorders, *see* Stuttering
Functional language use, 11–12, 51–52, 56, 63, 70, 108
assessment of, 75–82

G

Grammar, *see* Language structure

H

Hearing-impaired children, 12–13
tests for, 64–65
Home Bilingual Usage Estimate, 56

I

Identification of communicative disorders, 7–11
using published tests, 65–70
using nonstandardized measures, 87–88
Illinois Test of Psycholinguistic Abilities, 57
International registry, 27, 29
Interpreters, 17, 25, 26, 38–39, 42
training of, 18, 38–39
Interview techniques, 20
Inventories for communication assessment, 13, 98–100
pragmatic measures, 23–24, 78–81
questionnaires for parents, 56

J

James Language Dominance Test, 54, 55

L

Language
differences, 7–9, 58, 66, 107
disorders, 2, 7–11, 104
tests, 23, 54–63, 84–85
Language Assessment Scales, 55, 85, 122
Language dominance testing, 23, 54–56
Language environment, 7, 9, 11–12, 15, 27, 47–50, 58, 82
Language function, *see* Functional language use
Language of instruction, 104–107
Language loss, 9–10, 50
implications for assessment, 27
Language Modalities Test for Aphasia, 62
Language samples, *see* Samples of natural communication
Language structure,
analysis procedures, 82–83
developmental errors, 7–9
procedures for assessing, 51–52, 83–84
See also Discrete point tests
Least restrictive environment, 103–104
Linguistic borrowing, 10
Litigation, 1

M

Mean length of utterance, 82
Medida Española de Articulación, 53, 123
Minnesota Test for Differential Diagnosis of Aphasia, 62
Minority languages
structural descriptions of, 5, 59, 90–91, 93, 131–139

N

Native American cultures, 4, 44–45, 46
Needs assessment, 19–21
Nonstandardized assessment techniques, 13, 71–88
development of, 98–100
Nonverbal behaviors, 11, 44, 73
Normative data, 13, 57, 58
adequacy of, 66–67, 69
locally developed, 61, 67, 93, 95, 96–97
problems in using, 56–57, 60–61, 68
Norm-referenced language tests, 13, 56–61
construction of, 95–98
limitations of, 68–69, 87–88, 119
See also Assessment instruments
Northwestern Syntax Screen Test, 57

O

Observational assessment, 72–73
instruments for, 23–24, 78–82, 98–101
of child with peer group, 23–24, 72, 93, 99
techniques, 77–82

P

Paraprofessionals, 21, 26, 31–39, 42
as instructional resources, 109–110
as interpreters, 38–39
as referral sources, 37–38
as test administrators, 23, 26, 31, 35, 37
selection of, 36
training of, 26, 33–39, 109
Parents, 47, 107
as information sources, 81
as language models, 49
interviewing of, 39, 46–48, 111–112
roles in remedial programs, 108
Patterns of language use, 7, 14, 27
instruments for assessing, 48–49, 56
Patterns of support, 43–44
Peabody Picture Vocabulary Test, 57, 58, 91, 98
Phonological development
in first language, 5–6
in second language, 5–7
processes of, 6
Phonological processes, 4, 54, 94
Porch Index of Communicative Ability, 62
Poverty, 43–44, 47
Pragmatic referral criteria, 81
Program placement, 1, 103–104, 107–109
Pruebas de Expresión Oral y Percepción de la Lengua Española, 61, 114–115
Pruebas del Desarrollo Inicial del Lenguaje, 61, 113–114
Public Law 94-142, 1, 14, 18, 46, 51, 103

R

Referrals for assessment, 20, 21, 22–24, 37–38
appropriateness of, 22–23
pragmatic criteria and, 81
Reliability of tests, 56, 67, 92–93, 97
Remediation of communicative disorders
alternative placements for, 107–110
program eligibility for, 1, 22, 104

S

Samples of natural communication, 13, 18, 61
analysis of, 75
and handicap identification, 72
and language dominance assessment, 56
compared with tests, 69–70, 87–88, 97–98
contexts for, 74
procedures for collecting, 73–74
procedures for recording, 74–75
size of, 74
School records, 20
Screening for communicative disorders
classroom procedures for, 23–24, 37
pragmatic measures, 23–24
Screening Test of Spanish Grammar, 59, 61, 123
Second language acquisition
developmental sequences in, 7–8
handicap identification and, 1, 4–11
influence of first language on, 4–9
Sentence imitation, 84
Southwestern Spanish Articulation Test, 53, 123
Spanish
articulation tests, 53–54, 119–120, 123–124
language tests, 54–56, 59–61, 84–85, 113–125
Spanish Language Assessment Procedures, 85, 100, 124
Speech acts, 75, 100
recording of, 78
taxonomies of, 77–78
Speech discrimination testing, 64
Speech reception testing, 64
Spotting Language Problems, 81
Story contexts, 85–87
Stress patterns, 53, 64
Structural differences, 5–6, 93
and test translations, 58–60, 90
Structuralistic model of language, 51, 65
Structured language sampling, 83–84
Stuttering, 2, 3–4, 106

T

Teachers, 81, 99
  as referral sources, 81
  role in screening, 81
  training of, 21–22
Team approach, 14, 17–30, 32, 110
  and the assessment process, 17, 21–29
  and remedial program planning, 106
  and test construction, 95
  speech-language pathologist's role in, 17–18
  training for, 17–18, 21, 35–39
  use of community resources in, 24–25, 30
Templin-Darley Tests of Articulation, 52
Test content
  cultural appropriateness of, 66, 91–92
  development of, 95
  linguistic appropriateness of, 59, 66
  modification of, 91–93
Test evaluation, 65–67, 127–130
Test for Auditory Comprehension of Language, 57, 59, 124
Test of Early Language Development, 114
Test of Language Development, 78
Tests
  articulation, 23, 52–54
  criterion-referenced, 13, 61, 84–85, 98–100, 117–118
  discrete point, 51–56, 60
  guidelines for interpreting, 68–70
  language, 23, 54–63
  norm-referenced, 13, 56–61, 87–89, 95–98
  nonstandardized, 13, 71–88, 98–100
  See also Assessment instruments
Tone languages, 90–91
Toronto Tests of Receptive Vocabulary, 125
Translations of tests, 58–60, 90–91
Trochaic words, 64

V

Validity of tests, 55, 56, 59, 67, 91, 92–93, 97–98
Vietnamese culture, 44, 45, 81
Voice disorders, 2–3

W

Weiss Comprehensive Articulation Test, 53
Woodcock Language Proficiency Battery, 116
Woodcock Spanish Psycho-Educational Battery, 115–117
Word retrieval problems, 62